THE GOOD ENERGY COOKBOOK

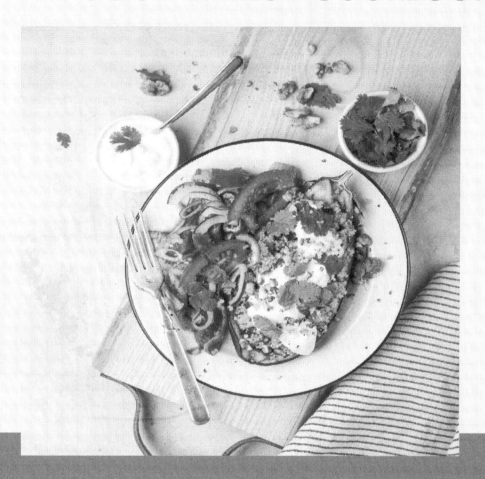

"Over 100 Low-Glycemic, Anti-Inflammatory Recipes to Boost Your Energy and Health.

Inspired by the experience of

Dr. Casey Means"

Nancy Johnson

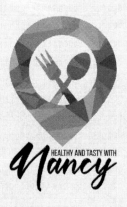

Table of Contents

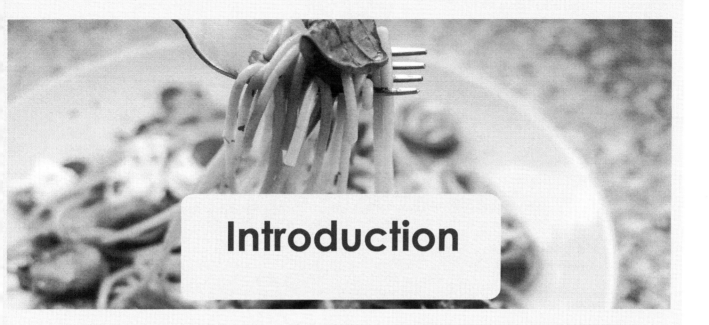

Introduction

EMBRACING GOOD ENERGY WITH DR. CASEY MEANS

Welcome to "The Good Energy Cookbook," a collection of recipes inspired by the insights and principles of Dr. Casey Means, a leading advocate for metabolic health and wellness. In this book, we aim to combine flavorful, nutrient-dense dishes with strategies to support your journey toward optimal health, energy, and well-being.

About dr. Casey means

Dr. Casey Means is a pioneering physician and a prominent advocate for using metabolic health to enhance overall wellness. With a background in both traditional medicine and cutting-edge nutritional science, Dr. Means has dedicated her career to exploring how metabolic health impacts energy levels, weight management, and disease prevention.

Dr. Means's approach is rooted in the understanding that maintaining balanced blood sugar levels and a healthy metabolism is crucial for achieving long-term health goals. Her work emphasizes the importance of integrating lifestyle changes, such as adopting a balanced diet, regular physical activity, and mindful stress management, to support metabolic health.

The philosophy behind the good energy cookbook

Inspired by Dr. Means's insights, "The Good Energy Cookbook" offers a selection of recipes designed to nourish your body, boost your energy, and support a balanced metabolism. Each recipe is crafted with a focus on whole, minimally processed ingredients that are rich in nutrients, fiber, and healthy fats while being low in refined sugars and unhealthy fats.Our goal is to provide you with practical, delicious meal options that not only satisfy your taste buds but also align with Dr. Means's principles of metabolic health. By incorporating these recipes into your daily routine, you'll be taking a proactive step toward managing your weight, improving your energy levels, and supporting overall health.

What to expect in this book

In this cookbook, you'll find a diverse array of recipes categorized to suit various meal times and dietary preferences:

- **Breakfast Recipes**: Start your day with energizing and satisfying options like Chia Seed Pudding with Fresh Berries and Apple Cinnamon Overnight Oats.

- **First Course Recipes**: Enjoy nutrient-rich soups and salads such as Spicy Moroccan Chickpea and Lentil Soup and Mediterranean Couscous Salad.

- **Meat Main Course Recipes**: Discover hearty and flavorful dishes like Spinach and Feta Stuffed Chicken Breast and Herbed Turkey Meatballs.

- **Fish-Based Main Course Recipes**: Delight in fresh, light meals including Grilled Salmon with Mango Salsa and Mediterranean Tuna Salad.

- **Side Dishes**: Complement your meals with wholesome sides like Sweet Potato and Kale Hash and Balsamic Glazed Brussels Sprouts.

- **Desserts**: Treat yourself to guilt-free indulgences such as Dark Chocolate Avocado Mousse and Baked Apples with Cinnamon and Walnuts.

How To Use This Book
Each recipe in this cookbook includes detailed preparation and cooking instructions, along with nutritional information to help you make informed choices. Whether you're looking to start your day on the right foot, enjoy a nourishing lunch, or prepare a satisfying dinner, the recipes here are designed to be both delicious and supportive of your health goals.

As you explore these recipes, remember that healthy eating is a journey, not a destination. It's about making small, sustainable changes that enhance your well-being and help you thrive. By integrating the principles of metabolic health into your daily life, you'll discover how nourishing your body with the right foods can transform your energy levels and overall health.

We hope this cookbook inspires you to embrace the power of good energy and embark on a path to a healthier, more vibrant you. Enjoy the journey and happy cooking!

Certainly! Let's continue with additional sections that provide further context and practical advice for using the cookbook:

GETTING STARTED WITH METABOLIC HEALTH
To fully benefit from the recipes in "The Good Energy Cookbook," it's helpful to understand some foundational concepts about metabolic health. Metabolism refers to the complex set of processes by which your body converts food into energy. A well-balanced metabolism supports stable blood sugar levels, efficient energy use, and overall well-being.

Dr. Casey Means emphasizes the importance of a balanced diet rich in whole foods that provide essential nutrients without causing blood sugar spikes. This includes incorporating:

- **Fiber-Rich Foods**: Such as vegetables, fruits, and whole grains, which help stabilize blood sugar levels and support digestion.

- **Healthy Fats**: Found in avocados, nuts, and olive oil, which provide sustained energy and support cellular health.

- **Lean Proteins**: Like chicken, fish, and legumes, which are crucial for muscle repair and energy maintenance.

NAVIGATING YOUR WAY THROUGH THE COOKBOOK

Here's a brief guide to help you navigate "The Good Energy Cookbook" effectively:

1. **Explore the Recipe Categories:** Start by browsing through the categories to find recipes that fit your current needs, whether you're looking for a quick breakfast, a hearty main course, or a satisfying dessert.

2. **Understand the Nutritional Information:** Each recipe includes detailed nutritional information to help you make informed choices. This includes calorie counts, protein, carbohydrate, fat content, and fiber. Use this information to balance your meals according to your personal health goals.

3. **Follow the Preparation Instructions:** The recipes are designed to be straightforward and manageable. Each one includes step-by-step instructions to ensure you can easily prepare and cook the dishes, even if you're new to cooking.

4. **Adapt Recipes to Your Preferences:** Feel free to modify ingredients based on your dietary preferences or restrictions. For example, substitute different vegetables or proteins based on what you have available or what you prefer.

5. **Incorporate These Meals into a Balanced Lifestyle:** While the recipes are designed to support metabolic health, combining them with regular physical activity, adequate hydration, and stress management will further enhance your overall well-being.

TIPS FOR SUCCESS

To make the most of the recipes in this cookbook, consider these practical tips:

- **Plan Your Meals:** Take some time each week to plan your meals. This will help you manage your grocery shopping and ensure you always have the ingredients you need on hand.

- **Prep in Advance:** Prepare ingredients or meals ahead of time to save time during busy days. For example, cook a batch of quinoa or roast vegetables in advance.

- **Stay Hydrated:** Drinking plenty of water throughout the day supports metabolic processes and overall health.

- **Listen to Your Body:** Pay attention to how different foods affect your energy levels and overall well-being. Adjust your diet based on what makes you feel your best.

A NOTE OF ENCOURAGEMENT

Embarking on a journey towards better health is a commendable decision. Remember, progress is achieved through consistent, small changes rather than drastic shifts. Celebrate each step you take towards a healthier lifestyle, and be patient with yourself as you make these changes.

We're excited for you to explore "The Good Energy Cookbook" and hope that the recipes and insights shared here inspire you to make nourishing choices that enhance your energy and well-being. Enjoy the journey towards a healthier, more vibrant you!

Happy cooking and best wishes for your health journey!

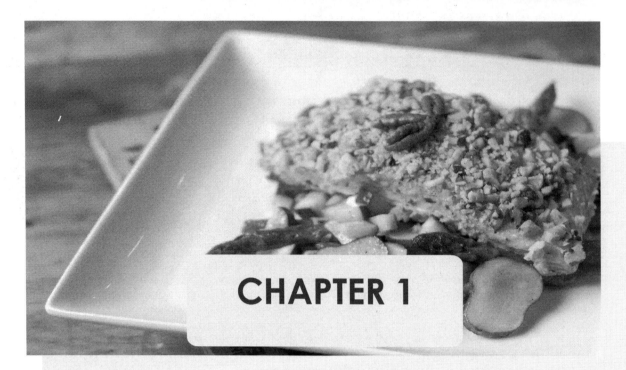

CHAPTER 1

The Foundations of an Anti-Inflammatory and Low Glycemic Index Diet

In recent years, the importance of nutrition in overall health and wellness has become increasingly clear. An anti-inflammatory and low glycemic index (GI) diet has emerged as one of the most effective approaches to achieving and maintaining optimal health. This chapter will delve into the principles of these diets, why they are crucial for sustainable wellness, and how they can be incorporated into everyday life to promote "good energy."

WHAT IS INFLAMMATION AND WHY DOES IT MATTER?

Inflammation is the body's natural response to injury, infection, or harmful stimuli. It is a protective mechanism that helps to heal wounds and fight infections. However, when inflammation becomes chronic, it can lead to a host of health problems, including obesity, diabetes, heart disease, autoimmune conditions, and even certain types of cancer. Chronic inflammation can be triggered by several factors, such as stress, lack of sleep, environmental toxins, and, importantly, diet. Foods high in refined sugars, trans fats, and artificial additives can contribute significantly to inflammation. Over time, this chronic inflammatory state can damage cells and tissues, disrupt normal bodily functions, and impair metabolic health.

THE ANTI-INFLAMMATORY DIET: A HOLISTIC APPROACH

An anti-inflammatory diet focuses on consuming foods that help reduce inflammation and avoiding those that trigger it. The principles are simple but profound:

1. Prioritize Whole, Unprocessed Foods: Fresh vegetables, fruits, nuts, seeds, lean proteins, and healthy fats form the basis of an anti-inflammatory diet. These foods are rich in antioxidants, vitamins, and minerals that help neutralize free radicals and reduce inflammation at the cellular level.

2. Choose Healthy Fats: Fats are not the enemy when it comes to inflammation. Instead, it's about choosing the right types of fats. Omega-3 fatty acids found in fatty fish (like salmon, sardines, and mackerel), chia seeds, flaxseeds, and walnuts have powerful anti-inflammatory effects. On the other hand, trans fats and excessive omega-6 fatty acids (found in many processed foods and certain vegetable oils) can exacerbate inflammation.

3. Embrace Anti-Inflammatory Herbs and Spices: Turmeric, ginger, garlic, cinnamon, and green tea are not only delicious but also packed with anti-inflammatory properties. These spices and herbs can help modulate inflammatory pathways and are an easy addition to meals.

4. Minimize Refined Sugars and Carbohydrates: High sugar intake has been linked to increased levels of inflammatory markers in the blood. Replacing refined sugars with natural alternatives like stevia, monk fruit, or raw honey, in moderation, can help mitigate these effects.

5. Avoid Processed and Packaged Foods: Many processed foods contain additives, preservatives, and artificial ingredients that can trigger inflammatory responses. Focus on cooking from scratch and using whole, natural ingredients to control what goes into your body.

UNDERSTANDING THE GLYCEMIC INDEX (GI)

The glycemic index (GI) is a ranking system for carbohydrates based on how they affect blood sugar levels. Foods with a high GI are quickly digested and absorbed, causing rapid spikes in blood sugar and insulin levels. Conversely, low-GI foods are digested and absorbed more slowly, resulting in a gradual rise in blood sugar and insulin levels. Maintaining stable blood sugar is crucial for preventing energy crashes, cravings, and long-term health issues like type 2 diabetes.

WHY A LOW GI DIET IS IMPORTANT

1. Stable Blood Sugar Levels: Low-GI foods help keep blood sugar levels stable, reducing the risk of insulin resistance, a precursor to diabetes and metabolic syndrome.

2. Better Weight Management: Low-GI foods tend to be more filling and provide sustained energy, which can help control appetite and prevent overeating.

3. Improved Energy and Mental Clarity: When blood sugar levels are stable, the body and brain receive a steady supply of energy, leading to better focus, mood, and cognitive function.

4. Lowered Risk of Chronic Diseases: A low-GI diet has been linked to a reduced risk of heart disease, certain cancers, and age-related eye diseases, among others.

COMBINING ANTI-INFLAMMATORY AND LOW GI PRINCIPLES

The magic happens when you combine an anti-inflammatory diet with a low-GI approach. Together, they provide a powerful framework for improving metabolic health, reducing chronic disease risk, and optimizing overall wellness.

- **Focus on Fiber-Rich Vegetables and Fruits:** Most vegetables and low-sugar fruits, like berries, are low on the glycemic index and rich in antioxidants, making them perfect choices for an anti-inflammatory diet.

- **Select Whole Grains Wisely:** Instead of refined grains, opt for low-GI whole grains like quinoa, barley, and steel-cut oats. These not only provide fiber and essential nutrients but also help maintain stable blood sugar levels.

- **Pair Proteins with Healthy Fats:** Proteins like fish, chicken, and legumes, when combined with healthy fats like olive oil, avocado, and nuts, create meals that are both anti-inflammatory and low GI.

- **Include Fermented Foods:** Foods like yogurt, kefir, sauerkraut, and kimchi not only support gut health but also help reduce inflammation.

- **Stay Hydrated:** Adequate hydration is essential for all bodily functions, including those that manage inflammation. Drinking enough water, herbal teas, and anti-inflammatory beverages like green tea can help maintain proper hydration levels.

PRACTICAL TIPS FOR EVERYDAY EATING

1. Meal Prep and Planning: Prepare meals ahead of time to ensure you have healthy, anti-inflammatory, and low-GI options readily available. This helps avoid the temptation of unhealthy, quick-fix meals.

2. Mindful Eating: Eat slowly and savor your food. This not only aids digestion but also helps you become more aware of hunger and fullness cues, preventing overeating.

3. Listen to Your Body: Everyone's body responds differently to certain foods. Use a food journal or consider continuous glucose monitoring (CGM) to understand how specific foods affect your blood sugar levels and overall well-being.

4. Experiment with Recipes: Use this cookbook as a foundation, but feel free to modify recipes to suit your taste and health goals. Swap ingredients, add anti-inflammatory spices, and try new combinations.

Adopting an anti-inflammatory, low-GI diet isn't about restriction but rather about choosing foods that nourish and energize the body. By focusing on these principles, you'll not only feel more energized but also take proactive steps toward preventing chronic diseases, managing your weight, and achieving overall wellness. In the following chapters, you'll find a variety of recipes crafted with these foundational principles in mind, designed to be delicious, nutritious, and aligned with your journey toward "good energy."

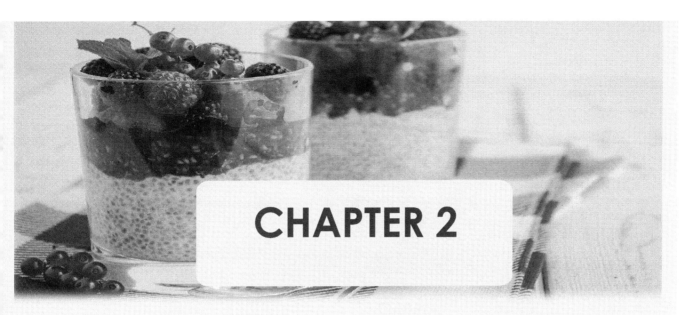

CHAPTER 2

Guide to Ingredients for Good Energy

Understanding the ingredients that fuel your body is the cornerstone of any successful wellness journey. In this chapter, we explore the key ingredients that not only provide essential nutrients but also help optimize energy levels, reduce inflammation, and promote overall well-being. These ingredients are carefully selected to align with the principles of an anti-inflammatory and low-glycemic index (GI) diet, ensuring that every meal contributes to sustained "good energy."

1. LEAFY GREENS

Leafy greens such as kale, spinach, Swiss chard, and arugula are foundational to any healthy diet. Rich in vitamins A, C, E, and K, as well as folate, iron, magnesium, potassium, and calcium, these greens provide essential nutrients while being incredibly low in calories.

- **Why They Matter:** Leafy greens are packed with antioxidants that help neutralize harmful free radicals in the body, reducing oxidative stress and inflammation. They are also a great source of fiber, aiding in digestion and helping to maintain stable blood sugar levels.

- **How to Use Them:** Incorporate leafy greens into smoothies, salads, soups, and sautés. Their versatility makes them easy to include in almost any meal.

2. HEALTHY FATS

Contrary to outdated dietary advice, healthy fats are vital for energy production, brain function, and overall health. Key sources include avocados, olive oil, nuts, seeds, and fatty fish like salmon, sardines, and mackerel.

- **Why They Matter:** Healthy fats, particularly omega-3 fatty acids, have powerful anti-inflammatory properties. They support heart health, improve cognitive function, and help maintain hormonal balance.

- **How to Use Them:** Use extra virgin olive oil as a base for salad dressings and marinades, add avocados to salads and sandwiches, and incorporate nuts and seeds into snacks and baked goods.

3. BERRIES

Berries such as blueberries, strawberries, raspberries, and blackberries are nutritional powerhouses. They are low in calories but high in fiber, vitamins, and antioxidants, particularly anthocyanins, which give them their vibrant color.

- **Why They Matter:** Berries have a low glycemic index, which means they don't cause rapid spikes in blood sugar. Their high antioxidant content helps combat inflammation and oxidative stress, promoting a healthy heart and brain.

- **How to Use Them:** Add berries to smoothies, yogurt, oatmeal, or salads, or enjoy them as a natural, low-sugar dessert.

4. WHOLE GRAINS AND LOW-GI CARBOHYDRATES

While refined carbohydrates can lead to inflammation and energy crashes, whole grains and low-GI carbs provide sustained energy without spiking blood sugar levels. Quinoa, barley, farro, steel-cut oats, and legumes are excellent choices.

- **Why They Matter:** These complex carbohydrates provide a slow release of energy, helping maintain stable blood sugar levels and reducing cravings. They are also high in fiber, which supports digestive health and promotes satiety.

- **How to Use Them:** Substitute refined grains with whole grains in recipes. Use quinoa or farro as a base for salads, add barley to soups, or start your day with a bowl of steel-cut oats.

5. FERMENTED FOODS

Fermented foods like yogurt, kefir, sauerkraut, kimchi, and miso are rich in probiotics, which are beneficial bacteria that support gut health.

- **Why They Matter:** A healthy gut microbiome is crucial for overall health, affecting everything from digestion and nutrient absorption to immunity and even mood regulation. Consuming fermented foods can help maintain a balanced gut microbiome, reduce inflammation, and improve metabolic health.

- **How to Use Them:** Add kimchi or sauerkraut to salads and sandwiches, use yogurt as a base for dressings and dips, or enjoy kefir as a smoothie base.

6. NUTS AND SEEDS

Almonds, walnuts, chia seeds, flaxseeds, pumpkin seeds, and sunflower seeds are nutrient-dense and packed with healthy fats, protein, fiber, and essential vitamins and minerals.

- **Why They Matter:** Nuts and seeds are anti-inflammatory and help regulate blood sugar levels. They are also rich in magnesium, which is essential for energy production and stress reduction.

- **How to Use Them:** Use them as a topping for salads, yogurt, or oatmeal, or blend them into smoothies. They also make great portable snacks.

7. LEAN PROTEINS

Protein is an essential macronutrient that plays a critical role in building and repairing tissues, producing enzymes and hormones, and supporting overall health. Lean protein sources include chicken, turkey, fish, tofu, tempeh, legumes, and beans.

- **Why They Matter:** Lean proteins are lower in saturated fats, helping to reduce inflammation and promote cardiovascular health. They also help regulate blood sugar levels by slowing the absorption of carbohydrates.

- How to Use Them: Grill or bake lean meats and fish, incorporate legumes and beans into soups and stews, or use tofu and tempeh in stir-fries and salads.

8. HERBS AND SPICES

Herbs and spices like turmeric, ginger, garlic, cinnamon, and rosemary not only enhance flavor but also offer powerful health benefits.

- Why They Matter: Many herbs and spices have potent anti-inflammatory and antioxidant properties. For example, curcumin in turmeric is known for its ability to reduce inflammation, while ginger helps with digestion and reduces nausea.

- How to Use Them: Add fresh herbs to salads and cooked dishes, use ground spices in soups, stews, and marinades, or make herbal teas.

9. HYDRATING FOODS AND BEVERAGES

Staying hydrated is essential for maintaining energy levels, supporting digestion, and reducing inflammation. Foods like cucumbers, watermelon, and citrus fruits, along with beverages like green tea, herbal infusions, and water with lemon, are excellent choices.

- Why They Matter: Proper hydration helps flush out toxins, supports kidney function, and maintains skin health. Green tea, for example, is rich in catechins, which are known for their anti-inflammatory and metabolism-boosting properties.

- How to Use Them: Start your day with a glass of water with lemon, drink green tea throughout the day, and snack on hydrating fruits and vegetables.

10. ANTI-INFLAMMATORY BEVERAGES

Beverages like green tea, herbal teas, and turmeric lattes not only provide hydration but also deliver powerful anti-inflammatory compounds.

- Why They Matter: These beverages help support a healthy metabolism, reduce oxidative stress, and promote calm and relaxation.

- How to Use Them: Replace sugary beverages with these anti-inflammatory options. A cup of green tea or a turmeric latte can also be a great way to start or end the day.

BUILDING YOUR PANTRY FOR GOOD ENERGY

A well-stocked pantry with these ingredients is the first step towards a sustainable lifestyle that promotes good energy and optimal health. By choosing nutrient-dense, anti-inflammatory, and low-GI foods, you create a solid foundation for your diet and well-being. This chapter serves as a guide to understanding the power of each ingredient and how it can be incorporated into delicious, health-boosting recipes. In the following chapters, you will find a variety of recipes that utilize these ingredients to help you achieve and maintain good energy every day.

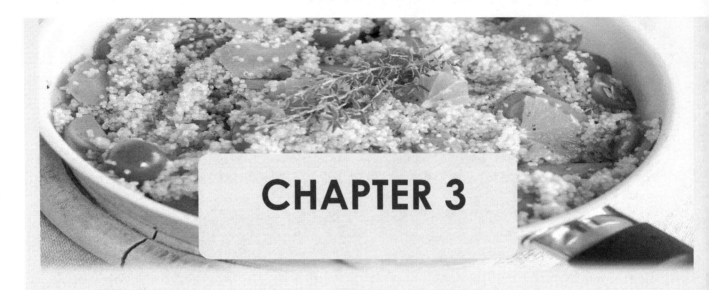

CHAPTER 3

Smart Meal Prep And Weekly Planning

Adopting a healthy lifestyle that aligns with an anti-inflammatory and low-glycemic diet requires more than just understanding what to eat; it involves strategic planning and preparation. "Smart Meal Prep" is about making healthy eating convenient, accessible, and sustainable, especially in today's busy world. This chapter provides you with practical tips, techniques, and strategies to effectively plan your meals for the week and execute them with ease, ensuring that you always have nutritious, energy-boosting food at your fingertips.

1. WHY MEAL PREP MATTERS

Meal prepping is the process of planning and preparing your meals in advance, usually for a few days or even an entire week. It is a powerful tool that supports a healthy diet and lifestyle for several reasons:

- **Saves Time and Reduces Stress:** Knowing what you'll eat ahead of time reduces the daily decision-making burden, saving you time and mental energy.

- **Supports Healthy Choices:** When you have pre-prepared meals and snacks, you're less likely to resort to unhealthy options, especially during busy or stressful times.

- **Portion Control:** Prepping meals in advance helps manage portion sizes, which is crucial for maintaining a healthy weight and stabilizing blood sugar levels.

- **Cost-Effective:** Meal prepping reduces food waste and minimizes the need for last-minute takeout or dining out, helping you stick to your budget.

- **Consistency:** A consistent approach to healthy eating ensures better energy levels, improved digestion, and overall well-being.

2. STEPS FOR EFFECTIVE WEEKLY MEAL PLANNING

A successful meal prep starts with a well-thought-out plan. Here's how to create a weekly meal plan that is both practical and nutritious:

1. **Assess Your Week:** Start by looking at your schedule for the week. Identify days when you'll have more time to cook and days when you'll need quick, ready-to-eat meals. Take note of any social events or commitments that may affect your meal times.

2. **Choose Your Recipes:** Select recipes that align with your dietary goals and are varied enough to keep your meals interesting. Aim for a balance of proteins, healthy fats, whole grains, and plenty of vegetables. Consider recipes that share similar ingredients to minimize waste and make shopping more efficient.

3. **Create a Shopping List:** Once you've chosen your recipes, make a comprehensive shopping list organized by sections of the grocery store (produce, grains, proteins, etc.). This will make your shopping trip faster and more efficient.

4. **Prep Smartly:** Designate a specific day for meal prep, such as Sunday or any day that suits your schedule. On this day, batch-cook grains, proteins, and vegetables that can be easily mixed and matched throughout the week. For example, cook a large batch of quinoa, roast a tray of mixed vegetables, and grill chicken breasts or tofu.

5. **Store Properly:** Use clear, BPA-free containers to store prepped ingredients and meals. Label each container with the contents and date to keep track of freshness. Store items like grains and proteins separately, so you can mix them up with different veggies and sauces for variety.

6. **Make Use of Freezer-Friendly Meals:** Some meals freeze well and can be a lifesaver on days when you have no time to cook. Soups, stews, and casseroles are great options to freeze in individual portions.

7. **Plan for Snacks and Beverages:** Don't forget to plan for snacks and drinks. Cut up veggies for easy snacking, portion out nuts and seeds, and prepare energy-boosting smoothies that can be stored in the fridge for a couple of days.

3. THE MEAL PREP ROUTINE: A STEP-BY-STEP GUIDE

Establishing a consistent meal prep routine can help you stick to your dietary goals. Here's a step-by-step guide to creating your own:

1. **Prep Breakfasts:** Focus on easy, grab-and-go options such as overnight oats, chia pudding, or egg muffins. These can be made in bulk and stored in the fridge or freezer.

2. **Cook Grains and Legumes in Batches:** Prepare a variety of grains like quinoa, brown rice, and farro, and legumes such as lentils and chickpeas. These serve as the base for many meals and can be easily stored in airtight containers.

3. **Prepare Proteins:** Grill, bake, or sauté proteins like chicken, tofu, tempeh, or fish in bulk. Keep seasoning simple and versatile so they can be used in a variety of dishes throughout the week.

4. **Chop Vegetables:** Pre-wash and chop vegetables for salads, stir-fries, and snacks. Store them in separate containers or bags in the fridge for quick access.

5. **Prepare Sauces and Dressings:** Homemade sauces and dressings not only taste better but are also healthier. Prepare a few versatile options like tahini dressing, lemon vinaigrette, or a simple olive oil and balsamic mix.

6. **Plan for Leftovers:** Purposefully cook extra portions of dinners that can be repurposed as lunch the next day. This reduces cooking time and ensures nothing goes to waste.

7. Reheat and Assemble: Each day, you can simply reheat and assemble your meals based on what you've prepped. Mix and match proteins, grains, and vegetables to keep things interesting.

4. TIPS FOR SMARTER MEAL PREP

To make meal prepping even more efficient and enjoyable, consider these additional tips:

- **Invest in Quality Storage Containers:** Good-quality containers will make your meal prep more effective. Look for ones that are airtight, dishwasher-safe, and BPA-free.

- **Use a Labeling System:** A simple labeling system will help you identify what needs to be consumed first, reducing waste.

- **Repurpose Ingredients:** Use ingredients in multiple ways. For example, grilled chicken can be used in salads, wraps, or paired with a side of veggies and grains.

- **Mix Up Flavors:** Use different spices, herbs, and sauces to give the same ingredients a new taste. This prevents meal fatigue and keeps your diet diverse.

- **Keep It Simple:** Start with basic recipes and gradually add variety. The more complex the plan, the less likely it is to stick. Simplicity is key.

5. SAMPLE WEEKLY MEAL PLAN

Here is a sample weekly meal plan that incorporates these meal prep strategies. This plan emphasizes variety and balance, focusing on anti-inflammatory, low-GI ingredients:

Day	Breakfast	Lunch	Dinner	Snack
Monday	Overnight oats with berries and chia seeds	Quinoa salad with chickpeas, roasted vegetables, and tahini dressing	Grilled salmon with steamed asparagus and sweet potato mash	Apple slices with almond butter
Tuesday	Green smoothie with spinach, avocado, and protein powder	Lentil soup with a side of mixed green salad	Tofu stir-fry with broccoli, bell peppers, and brown rice	Carrot and cucumber sticks with hummus
Wednesday	Chia seed pudding with coconut milk and mango	Chicken and quinoa bowl with kale, avocado, and lemon vinaigrette	Baked cod with roasted Brussels sprouts and cauliflower rice	Mixed nuts and seeds

A FOUNDATION FOR SUCCESS

By adopting a smart meal prep strategy, you set the foundation for consistent healthy eating, even on the busiest days. With just a few hours of planning and preparation each week, you can ensure that nutritious, delicious, and energy-boosting meals are always within reach. Use this chapter as a guide to establish your own meal prep routine, tailored to your needs and lifestyle, and enjoy the benefits of a more organized, stress-free approach to healthy living.

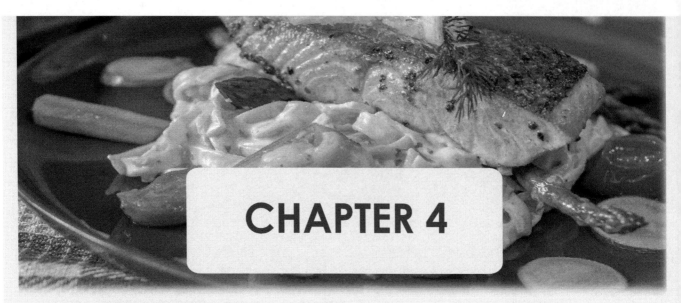

CHAPTER 4

Mindfulness Strategies and Conscious Eating

In a world where we often eat on the go, multitask during meals, or mindlessly snack in front of screens, the concept of mindful eating can feel like a breath of fresh air. Mindfulness, the practice of being fully present in the moment without judgment, can be a powerful tool when applied to eating habits. This chapter explores how mindfulness and conscious eating can transform not only your relationship with food but also your overall well-being. By developing a deeper awareness of what, why, and how you eat, you can foster a healthier, more balanced approach to nutrition and life.

1. THE IMPORTANCE OF MINDFUL EATING

Mindful eating is not about dieting or restricting food; it is about paying attention to the eating experience in a holistic and compassionate way. Here's why it matters:

- **Enhances Digestion:** Eating slowly and chewing thoroughly can improve digestion by giving your stomach time to signal fullness, reducing the likelihood of overeating.

- **Reduces Emotional Eating:** Mindful eating helps you distinguish between true hunger and emotional cravings, allowing you to address emotional needs in healthier ways.

- **Promotes Healthy Weight Management:** By focusing on the experience of eating, people often find they eat less and feel more satisfied, contributing to healthier weight management.

- **Builds a Positive Relationship with Food:** Instead of labeling foods as "good" or "bad," mindful eating encourages a more balanced and non-judgmental approach to all types of food.

- **Increases Gratitude and Enjoyment:** Mindfulness brings a sense of appreciation for the flavors, textures, and nourishment that food provides, turning meals into a more enjoyable and fulfilling experience.

2. PRINCIPLES OF MINDFUL EATING

Mindful eating revolves around several key principles that guide how we think about and interact with food:

1. Eat Without Distractions: Set aside time to eat without multitasking. This means turning off the TV, putting away your phone, and focusing solely on your meal.

2. Listen to Your Body: Recognize hunger and fullness cues. Eat when you're truly hungry and stop when you're comfortably satisfied, not overly full.

3. Savor Each Bite: Pay attention to the taste, texture, and aroma of your food. Take smaller bites and chew slowly, allowing your taste buds to fully experience the flavors.

4. Acknowledge Emotional Triggers: Notice if you are eating out of boredom, stress, or sadness rather than physical hunger. Developing this awareness helps you make more intentional food choices.

5. Practice Gratitude: Before eating, take a moment to express gratitude for the food, the effort that went into preparing it, and the nourishment it provides. This can shift your mindset to a more positive and mindful state.

3. MINDFUL EATING TECHNIQUES

To cultivate mindful eating habits, consider incorporating the following techniques into your daily routine:

1. The "Five Senses" Exercise: Engage all five senses while eating. Notice the colors and presentation of the food (sight), listen to the sounds of preparation or crunching (sound), inhale the aroma (smell), feel the textures with your hands or tongue (touch), and finally, savor the taste (taste). This exercise deepens your awareness and enjoyment of the meal.

2. The "Pause and Reflect" Method: Before each meal, take a few deep breaths and check in with yourself. Are you feeling hungry, tired, stressed, or anxious? Recognizing your emotional state can help prevent mindless eating and encourage more conscous choices.

3. Mindful Portion Control: Instead of piling your plate high, start with smaller portions. You can always take more if you're still hungry. This helps prevent overeating and encourages you to savor each bite.

4. The "Eating Meditation": Choose a simple food, such as a raisin or a piece of fruit, and eat it as if you've never tasted it before. Focus on every aspect of the experience, from picking it up to swallowing it. This practice enhances your ability to focus and appreciate food.

5. Set a Mealtime Ritual: Establish a calming routine before meals, such as lighting a candle, playing soft music, or practicing deep breathing exercises. A ritual can set a mindful tone and make eating a more intentional act.

4. INCORPORATING MINDFULNESS INTO DAILY MEALS

Integrating mindfulness into your daily eating routine doesn't have to be complicated. Here are some practical ways to get started:

- **Start with Breakfast:** Take a few moments to sit down and enjoy your breakfast without rushing. Even if it's just 10 minutes, use this time to practice mindful eating.

- **Mindful Lunch Breaks:** If possible, step away from your workspace or daily activities to eat lunch. Focus on the food and the break it provides from the hustle and bustle.

- **End the Day Mindfully:** Dinner is a great opportunity to reflect on the day and wind down. Make it a screen-free meal and take time to enjoy the flavors and nourishment.

- **Mindful Snacking:** When you feel the urge to snack, ask yourself if you're truly hungry or if it's a habit or emotional craving. If you are hungry, choose a snack that satisfies both your taste buds and nutritional needs.

5. THE CONNECTION BETWEEN MINDFULNESS AND NUTRITION

Mindfulness isn't just about the act of eating; it also extends to understanding the nutritional value and source of your food. When you eat mindfully, you become more aware of how certain foods make you feel—energized, sluggish, satisfied, or hungry. This awareness can guide you in making choices that are more aligned with your health goals.

- **Recognize the Impact of Ingredients:** Pay attention to how different foods affect your body. Foods high in sugar might cause a quick energy spike followed by a crash, while whole grains and proteins provide more sustained energy.

- **Mindful Cooking:** Engage in mindful practices while preparing meals. Chop vegetables with intention, breathe deeply as you cook, and consider the health benefits of the ingredients you're using.

- **Reflect on Your Food Choices:** After meals, take a moment to reflect on how the food made you feel. Did it nourish your body and mind? Did it satisfy your hunger? This reflection helps you become more attuned to your body's needs.

6. BENEFITS OF COMBINING MINDFULNESS AND ANTI-INFLAMMATORY EATING

Combining mindfulness with an anti-inflammatory, low-glycemic diet can amplify the benefits of both practices. Here's how they complement each other:

- **Improved Digestion and Metabolism:** Mindful eating encourages thorough chewing and slower eating, which aids digestion and supports a healthy metabolism.

- **Balanced Blood Sugar Levels:** A mindful approach to choosing low-glycemic foods helps maintain stable blood sugar levels, reducing cravings and mood swings.

- **Reduced Stress and Inflammation:** Mindfulness practices, like deep breathing and meditation, help manage stress, which is a significant contributor to inflammation.

- **Enhanced Body Awareness:** Mindful eating fosters a deeper connection with your body, helping you make food choices that reduce inflammation and boost energy.

A JOURNEY TO CONSCIOUS LIVING

Mindfulness and conscious eating are not about perfection; they are about progress. The journey toward mindful eating is one of self-awareness, compassion, and intentional choices. By incorporating these practices into your daily routine, you can develop a more balanced relationship with food, enhance your overall well-being, and fully embrace a healthier lifestyle.

Start small, be patient with yourself, and remember that every mindful moment you create around food brings you closer to a more harmonious and energized life.

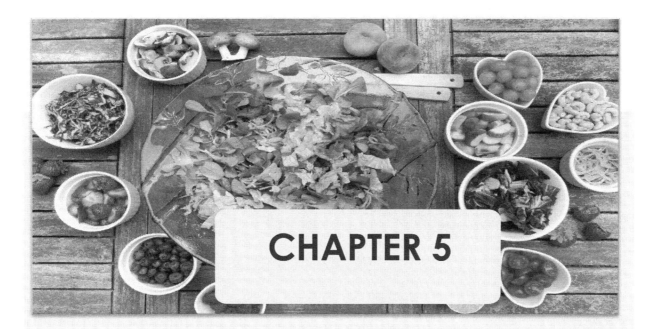

CHAPTER 5

Holistic Support for Well-Being

In our pursuit of optimal health, it's easy to focus solely on diet and exercise, but true well-being encompasses a broader range of factors. Holistic support for well-being takes into account the interconnectedness of body, mind, and spirit, emphasizing that each component plays a crucial role in achieving overall health. This chapter delves into the principles of holistic well-being and offers practical strategies to foster a balanced, healthy lifestyle.

1. UNDERSTANDING HOLISTIC WELL-BEING

Holistic well-being is a comprehensive approach that addresses the physical, emotional, mental, and spiritual aspects of health. Rather than viewing health as merely the absence of illness, a holistic perspective recognizes that true well-being arises from a harmonious balance between all these facets of life. Here's what this means in practice:

- **Physical Health:** This includes proper nutrition, regular exercise, adequate sleep, and routine medical care. It's the foundation upon which other aspects of well-being are built.

- **Emotional Health:** Emotional well-being involves understanding, managing, and expressing emotions in a healthy way. It includes building strong relationships, practicing self-care, and seeking support when needed.

- **Mental Health:** Mental well-being refers to cognitive and psychological aspects, such as managing stress, cultivating resilience, and engaging in activities that stimulate the mind.

- **Spiritual Health:** Spiritual well-being is about finding purpose, meaning, and connection. It doesn't necessarily mean religious practice but involves exploring your values, beliefs, and sense of inner peace.

2. THE INTERCONNECTEDNESS OF HEALTH

The components of holistic well-being are deeply interconnected. For example:

- **Physical Activity and Mental Health:** Regular exercise not only improves physical fitness but also releases endorphins that enhance mood and reduce anxiety.

- **Nutrition and Emotional Well-Being:** A balanced diet supports brain function and regulates mood. Nutrient-rich foods can help stabilize emotions and improve overall mental health.

- **Sleep and Cognitive Function:** Quality sleep is crucial for cognitive processes, memory consolidation, and emotional regulation. Poor sleep can lead to decreased mental clarity and increased stress levels.

- **Mindfulness and Spiritual Growth:** Mindfulness practices, such as meditation and reflection, can enhance spiritual awareness and foster a sense of inner calm and purpose.

3. PRACTICAL STRATEGIES FOR HOLISTIC WELL-BEING

To support a holistic approach to well-being, consider incorporating the following practices into your daily routine:

1. **Balanced Nutrition:** Focus on a varied diet rich in whole foods, including fruits, vegetables, lean proteins, and healthy fats. Avoid excessive processed foods and sugars that can disrupt physical and emotional balance.

2. **Regular Exercise:** Engage in physical activity that you enjoy, whether it's walking, yoga, swimming, or strength training. Aim for at least 150 minutes of moderate exercise per week, as recommended by health guidelines.

3. **Quality Sleep:** Establish a consistent sleep routine by going to bed and waking up at the same time each day. Create a restful environment and limit exposure to screens before bedtime to improve sleep quality.

4. **Emotional Expression:** Practice emotional self-care by expressing feelings through journaling, talking with a friend, or seeking professional counseling. Building supportive relationships and having outlets for emotional expression can enhance well-being.

5. **Mental Stimulation:** Keep your mind active by engaging in intellectually stimulating activities, such as reading, puzzles, or learning a new skill. Mental challenges can boost cognitive function and creativity.

6. **Mindfulness and Meditation:** Incorporate mindfulness practices into your daily routine. Spend a few minutes each day meditating, practicing deep breathing, or engaging in mindful activities to reduce stress and increase self-awareness.

7. **Spiritual Exploration:** Explore your personal values, beliefs, and sense of purpose. Whether through religious practices, philosophical exploration, or connecting with nature, find ways to nurture your spiritual well-being.

8. **Self-Care Rituals:** Create self-care routines that nurture your body, mind, and spirit. This might include relaxing baths, creative hobbies, or time spent in nature. Regular self-care helps maintain balance and rejuvenation.

4. BUILDING A HOLISTIC SUPPORT NETWORK

Having a strong support network is an essential part of holistic well-being. Surround yourself with people who encourage and uplift you, and don't hesitate to seek professional support when needed. Consider the following:

- **Health Professionals:** Regular check-ups with healthcare providers ensure that physical health is monitored and maintained. Consult with dietitians, therapists, or fitness experts for personalized advice.

- **Support Groups:** Join groups or communities that align with your interests or health goals. Being part of a supportive network can provide motivation and reduce feelings of isolation.

- **Family and Friends:** Cultivate relationships with people who offer emotional support and encouragement. Share your well-being goals and seek their understanding and involvement.

5. THE ROLE OF SELF-REFLECTION

Self-reflection is a key component of holistic well-being. Regularly assess your physical, emotional, mental, and spiritual health to identify areas for improvement and growth. Ask yourself:

- **Physical Health:** Am I meeting my nutritional and fitness goals? How is my energy level?

- **Emotional Health:** How am I managing stress and emotions? Do I feel supported by my relationships?

- **Mental Health:** Am I engaging in activities that challenge and stimulate my mind? How is my mental clarity?

- **Spiritual Health:** Do I feel a sense of purpose and connection? How can I deepen my spiritual practices?

EMBRACING HOLISTIC WELL-BEING

Embracing a holistic approach to well-being means acknowledging that health is a multifaceted journey, not a destination. By addressing the interconnected aspects of physical, emotional, mental, and spiritual health, you can create a more balanced and fulfilling life. Integrate these practices into your daily routine, and remember that well-being is an ongoing process of growth and self-discovery. By supporting yourself holistically, you empower yourself to lead a vibrant and enriched life.

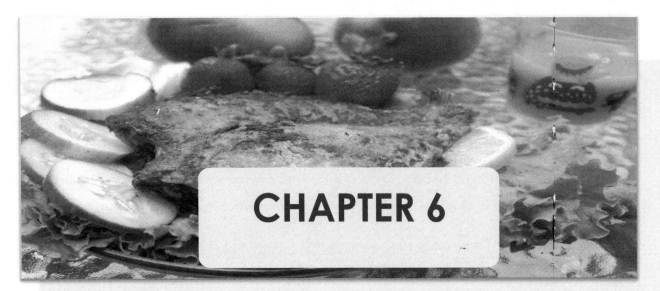

CHAPTER 6

Personalized Diet with Continuous Glucose Monitoring (CGM)

In the pursuit of a more tailored approach to health and nutrition, Continuous Glucose Monitoring (CGM) offers an innovative solution. This technology, traditionally used for managing diabetes, has increasingly become a valuable tool for anyone seeking to optimize their diet and well-being. This chapter explores how CGM works, its benefits for personalized nutrition, and practical steps for incorporating it into your lifestyle.

1. UNDERSTANDING CONTINUOUS GLUCOSE MONITORING (CGM)

Continuous Glucose Monitoring (CGM) is a technology that provides real-time insights into glucose levels in the body. It involves a small sensor placed under the skin, typically on the abdomen or arm, which continuously measures glucose levels in the interstitial fluid (the fluid between cells). The sensor transmits this data to a receiver or smartphone app, allowing users to monitor their glucose levels throughout the day.

Key Components of CGM:

- **Sensor:** A small device inserted just under the skin that measures glucose levels.

- **Transmitter:** A component that sends the glucose data from the sensor to a receiver or smartphone app.

- **Receiver/Smartphone App:** Displays the glucose data in real-time, providing insights into fluctuations and trends.

2. BENEFITS OF CGM FOR PERSONALIZED NUTRITION

Using CGM for personalized nutrition offers several benefits:

- **Real-Time Insights:** CGM provides continuous, real-time data on glucose levels, allowing you to understand how your body responds to different foods, meals, and activities.

- **Identifying Patterns:** By tracking glucose levels over time, CGM helps identify patterns and trends, such as how specific foods or meals impact your glucose levels and overall energy.

- **Improving Dietary Choices:** With real-time feedback, you can make more informed decisions about your diet, choosing foods that stabilize glucose levels and avoid those that cause spikes or crashes.

- **Enhanced Metabolic Health:** Maintaining stable glucose levels can improve metabolic health, reducing the risk of developing insulin resistance, type 2 diabetes, and other related conditions.

- **Personalized Feedback:** CGM offers personalized insights tailored to your unique physiological responses, allowing for a customized approach to nutrition and well-being.

3. HOW TO USE CGM FOR PERSONALIZED DIET

Integrating CGM into your dietary routine involves several steps:

1. Selecting a CGM System: Choose a CGM system that fits your needs and preferences. Consult with a healthcare professional to determine the best option for you.

2. Setting Up the Sensor: Follow the manufacturer's instructions to insert and set up the CGM sensor. Ensure the sensor is properly positioned and calibrated for accurate readings.

3. Monitoring Glucose Levels: Use the receiver or smartphone app to monitor your glucose levels throughout the day. Pay attention to trends and fluctuations, and note how they correlate with different foods and activities.

4. Analyzing Data: Review the data regularly to identify patterns and insights. Look for trends, such as glucose spikes after specific meals or drops in energy levels.

5. Adjusting Your Diet: Based on the insights gained from CGM data, adjust your dietary choices to maintain stable glucose levels. Opt for foods that have a minimal impact on glucose levels and experiment with different meal timings and compositions.

6. Incorporating Feedback: Use the data to fine-tune your diet and lifestyle. For example, if you notice that a particular snack causes a significant glucose spike, consider substituting it with a healthier option.

7. Consulting with Professionals: Regularly consult with a healthcare provider or dietitian to interpret CGM data and receive personalized recommendations. They can help you understand the implications of your glucose patterns and guide you in making dietary adjustments.

4. PRACTICAL TIPS FOR USING CGM EFFECTIVELY

To make the most of your CGM experience, consider these practical tips:

- **Keep a Food Diary:** Track your food intake alongside CGM data to see how different foods affect your glucose levels. This can help identify which foods are beneficial or problematic.

- **Monitor Physical Activity:** Note how exercise impacts your glucose levels. Physical activity can influence glucose metabolism and help stabilize levels.

- **Stay Hydrated:** Proper hydration can affect glucose levels. Ensure you drink enough water throughout the day.

- **Be Mindful of Stress:** Stress can influence glucose levels. Incorporate stress-reducing techniques, such as mindfulness or relaxation exercises, to maintain stable glucose levels.

- **Adjust Meal Timing:** Experiment with meal timing and frequency. Some people find that eating smaller, more frequent meals helps stabilize glucose levels, while others may benefit from intermittent fasting.

5. THE FUTURE OF PERSONALIZED NUTRITION WITH CGM

As technology advances, the use of CGM for personalized nutrition is likely to become even more sophisticated. Future developments may include:

- **Advanced Algorithms:** Improved algorithms that provide more precise recommendations based on individual glucose patterns and lifestyle factors.

- **Integration with Other Technologies:** Enhanced integration with other health technologies, such as wearable fitness trackers and health apps, for a more comprehensive view of well-being.

- **Expanded Accessibility:** Greater availability of CGM systems and reduced costs, making personalized nutrition more accessible to a broader audience.

EMBRACING CGM FOR PERSONALIZED NUTRITION

Continuous Glucose Monitoring (CGM) offers a powerful tool for personalized nutrition, providing real-time insights into how your body responds to different foods and activities. By leveraging CGM data, you can make more informed dietary choices, enhance metabolic health, and achieve a more tailored approach to well-being. Embrace this technology as part of your holistic health journey, and enjoy the benefits of a personalized, data-driven approach to nutrition.

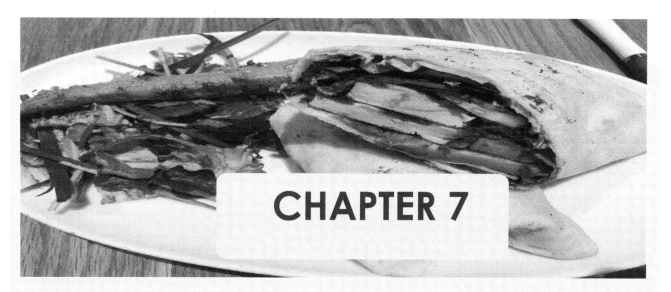

CHAPTER 7

Recipes 100+

1. AVOCADO & CHICKPEA SALAD WRAP

 Servings: 04   **Prep. time:** 15 minutes   **Cook time:** 10 minutes

INGREDIENTS

- 1 ripe avocado, mashed
- 1 cup cooked chickpeas
(canned, drained, and rinsed)
- 1/4 cup plain Greek yogurt
- 1 tablespoon lemon juice
- 1 tablespoon olive oil
- 1 teaspoon ground cumin
- Salt and pepper to taste
- 1 cup fresh spinach
- 1/2 cup shredded carrots
- 1/2 cup sliced cucumber
- 4 whole wheat tortillas

INSTRUCTIONS

1. In a medium bowl, mash the avocado until creamy. Add the chickpeas, Greek yogurt, lemon juice, olive oil, cumin, salt, and pepper. Mix well until the ingredients are well combined.
2. Spread the avocado and chickpea mixture onto each whole wheat tortilla.
3. Add a handful of spinach, shredded carrots, and sliced cucumber.
4. Roll up the tortillas and cut them in half.
5. Serve immediately or store in the refrigerator for up to 2 days.

Nutritional Information (per serving):- Calories: 250- Protein: 8g- Carbohydrates: 30g- Fat: 12g- Fiber: 8g

Servings: 04

Prep. time: 15 minutes

Cook time: 10 minutes

INGREDIENTS

- 1 head of cauliflower, grated into "rice"

- 2 tablespoons coconut oil

- 1 red onion, thinly sliced

- 2 garlic cloves, minced

- 1 red bell pepper, sliced

- 1 cup broccoli, cut into small pieces

- 1 teaspoon fresh ginger, grated

- 2 tablespoons low-sodium soy sauce

- 1 teaspoon sesame oil

- 1 tablespoon sesame seeds

- 1 teaspoon red pepper flakes (optional)

- 2 green onions, sliced for garnish

INSTRUCTIONS

1. In a medium bowl, mash the avocado until creamy. Add the chickpeas, Greek yogurt, lemon juice, olive oil, cumin, salt, and pepper. Mix well until the ingredients are well combined.

2. Spread the avocado and chickpea mixture onto each whole wheat tortilla.

3. Add a handful of spinach, shredded carrots, and sliced cucumber.

4. Roll up the tortillas and cut them in half.

5. Serve immediately or store in the refrigerator for up to 2 days.

Nutritional Information (per serving):- Calories: 250- Protein: 8g- Carbohydrates: 30g- Fat: 12g- Fiber: 8g

3. CHIA PUDDING WITH MIXED BERRIES

Servings: 02

Prep. time: 05 minutes

Cook time: 00 minutes

INGREDIENTS

- 1/4 cup chia seeds
- 1 cup unsweetened almond milk
- 1 teaspoon vanilla extract
- 1 tablespoon pure maple syrup
- 1/2 cup fresh strawberries, sliced
- 1/2 cup fresh blueberries
- 1/4 cup fresh raspberries
- 1 tablespoon sliced almonds (optional)

INSTRUCTIONS

1. In a medium bowl, combine the chia seeds, almond milk, vanilla extract, and maple syrup. Mix well until the chia seeds are evenly distributed.
2. Cover the bowl with plastic wrap and place it in the refrigerator for at least 4 hours or overnight, until the mixture thickens and resembles pudding.
3. Before serving, divide the chia pudding into bowls or dessert glasses and top with strawberries, blueberries, raspberries, and sliced almonds.
4. Serve chilled.

Nutritional Information (per serving): - Calories: 290- Protein: 10g- Carbohydrates: 40g- Fat: 8g- Fiber: 8g

4. QUINOA AND VEGGIE STUFFED BELL PEPPERS

Servings: 02   **Prep. time:** 05 minutes   **Cook time:** 00 minutes

INGREDIENTS

- 4 bell peppers (any color), tops cut off and seeds removed

- 1 cup quinoa, rinsed

- 2 cups vegetable broth

- 1 tablespoon olive oil

- 1 small onion, diced

- 2 garlic cloves, minced

- 1 zucchini, diced

- 1 cup cherry tomatoes, halved

- 1 cup black beans, rinsed and drained

- 1 teaspoon cumin

- 1 teaspoon smoked paprika

- Salt and pepper to taste

- 1/2 cup shredded low-fat cheddar cheese (optional)

- Fresh cilantro for garnish

INSTRUCTIONS

1. Preheat the oven to 375°F (190°C). Arrange the bell peppers in a baking dish.

2. In a medium saucepan, combine quinoa and vegetable broth. Bring to a boil, reduce heat, cover, and simmer for 15 minutes or until quinoa is fluffy.

3. In a large skillet, heat olive oil over medium heat. Add onion and garlic, and sauté for 2-3 minutes until softened.

4. Add zucchini and cherry tomatoes, and cook for 5 minutes until tender.

5. Stir in the cooked quinoa, black beans, cumin, smoked paprika, salt, and pepper. Cook for another 2-3 minutes until well combined.

6. Spoon the quinoa mixture into each bell pepper, filling them completely.

7. If desired, sprinkle shredded cheddar cheese on top of each pepper.

8. Cover the dish with foil and bake for 30 minutes. Remove the foil and bake for an additional 10 minutes until the peppers are tender and the cheese is melted and bubbly.

9. Garnish with fresh cilantro and serve warm.

Nutritional Information (per serving): - Calories: 290- Protein: 10g- Carbohydrates: 40g- Fat: 8g- Fiber: 8g

Servings: 04   **Prep. time:** 15 minutes   **Cook time:** 15 minutes

INGREDIENTS

- 4 medium zucchinis, spiralized into noodles

- 2 tablespoons olive oil, divided

- 2 chicken breasts, boneless and skinless

- Salt and pepper to taste

- 1 cup fresh basil leaves

- 1/4 cup pine nuts, toasted

- 2 garlic cloves

- 1/4 cup Parmesan cheese, grated

- 1/4 cup olive oil

- 1 tablespoon lemon juice

INSTRUCTIONS

1. Heat 1 tablespoon of olive oil in a large skillet over medium-high heat. Season chicken breasts with salt and pepper. Grill the chicken in the skillet for 6-7 minutes per side, or until fully cooked. Let it rest for a few minutes before slicing.
2. In a food processor, combine basil leaves, toasted pine nuts, garlic, Parmesan cheese, and lemon juice. Pulse until finely chopped.
3. With the processor running, slowly add 1/4 cup of olive oil until the mixture is smooth and creamy. Season with salt and pepper.
4. In the same skillet, add the remaining 1 tablespoon of olive oil and sauté the zucchini noodles for 2-3 minutes until just tender.
5. Toss the zucchini noodles with the pesto sauce until well coated.
6. Divide the noodles into bowls, top with sliced grilled chicken, and serve immediately.

Nutritional Information (per serving):- Calories: 350- Protein: 28g- Carbohydrates: 10g- Fat: 23g- Fiber: 4g

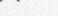

Servings: 01

Prep. time: 5 minutes (+ overnight soaking)

Cook time: 00 minutes

INGREDIENTS

- 4 medium zucchinis, spiralized into noodles

- 2 tablespoons olive oil, divided

- 2 chicken breasts, boneless and skinless

- Salt and pepper to taste

- 1 cup fresh basil leaves

- 1/4 cup pine nuts, toasted

- 2 garlic cloves

- 1/4 cup Parmesan cheese, grated

- 1/4 cup olive oil

- 1 tablespoon lemon juice

INSTRUCTIONS

1. Heat 1 tablespoon of olive oil in a large skillet over medium-high heat. Season chicken breasts with salt and pepper. Grill the chicken in the skillet for 6-7 minutes per side, or until fully cooked. Let it rest for a few minutes before slicing.
2. In a food processor, combine basil leaves, toasted pine nuts, garlic, Parmesan cheese, and lemon juice. Pulse until finely chopped.
3. With the processor running, slowly add 1/4 cup of olive oil until the mixture is smooth and creamy. Season with salt and pepper.
4. In the same skillet, add the remaining 1 tablespoon of olive oil and sauté the zucchini noodles for 2-3 minutes until just tender.
5. Toss the zucchini noodles with the pesto sauce until well coated.
6. Divide the noodles into bowls, top with sliced grilled chicken, and serve immediately.

Nutritional Information (per serving):- Calories: 350- Protein: 28g- Carbohydrates: 10g- Fat: 23g- Fiber: 4g

Servings: 04   **Prep. time:** 10 minutes   **Cook time:** 25 minutes

INGREDIENTS

- 2 medium sweet potatoes, peeled and diced

- 2 tablespoons olive oil

- 1 teaspoon chili powder

- 1 teaspoon cumin

- Salt and pepper to taste

- 1 can (15 oz) black beans, drained and rinsed

- 8 small corn tortillas

- 1/2 cup red cabbage, shredded

- 1/2 cup diced avocado

- 1/4 cup chopped fresh cilantro

- 2 tablespoons lime juice

- 1/4 cup Greek yogurt or sour cream (optional)

INSTRUCTIONS

1. Preheat the oven to 425°F (220°C). On a baking sheet, toss the diced sweet potatoes with olive oil, chili powder, cumin, salt, and pepper. Roast for 20-25 minutes, stirring halfway through, until tender and slightly crispy.

2. In a small saucepan over medium heat, warm the black beans for 5 minutes until heated through.

3. Warm the corn tortillas in a dry skillet or microwave.

4. Assemble the tacos by layering roasted sweet potatoes, black beans, shredded red cabbage, diced avocado, and a sprinkle of fresh cilantro.

5. Drizzle with lime juice and add a dollop of Greek yogurt or sour cream, if desired.

6. Serve immediately.

Nutritional Information (per serving):- Calories: 280- Protein: 7g- Carbohydrates: 40g- Fat: 11g- Fiber: 10g

8. LENTIL AND VEGETABLE SOUP

Servings: 06   **Prep. time:** 15 minutes   **Cook time:** 35 minutes

INGREDIENTS

- 1 tablespoon olive oil

- 1 large onion, diced

- 3 garlic cloves, minced

- 2 carrots, diced

- 2 celery stalks, diced

- 1 cup dried lentils, rinsed

- 4 cups vegetable broth

- 1 can (14.5 oz) diced tomatoes

- 1 teaspoon dried thyme

- 1/2 teaspoon dried rosemary

- Salt and pepper to taste

- 2 cups fresh spinach, roughly chopped

- 1 tablespoon lemon juice

INSTRUCTIONS

1. In a large pot, heat olive oil over medium heat. Add the onion, garlic, carrots, and celery. Sauté for 5-7 minutes until softened.
2. Add the lentils, vegetable broth, diced tomatoes, thyme, rosemary, salt, and pepper. Bring to a boil.
3. Reduce heat, cover, and simmer for 25-30 minutes, or until the lentils are tender.
4. Stir in the spinach and cook for an additional 5 minutes until wilted.
5. Add lemon juice and adjust seasoning as needed.
6. Serve hot with whole-grain bread or a side salad.

Nutritional Information (per serving):- Calories: 210- Protein: 12g- Carbohydrates: 35g- Fat: 12g- Fiber: 12g

Servings: 04   **Prep. time:** 15 minutes   **Cook time:** 00 minutes

INGREDIENTS

- 1 can (15 oz) chickpeas, drained and rinsed

- 1 cup cherry tomatoes, halved

- 1 cucumber, diced

- 1/2 red onion, finely diced

- 1/2 cup Kalamata olives, pitted and sliced

- 1/4 cup crumbled feta cheese

- 2 tablespoons chopped fresh parsley

- 2 tablespoons extra virgin olive oil

- 1 tablespoon red wine vinegar

- 1 teaspoon dried oregano

- Salt and pepper to taste

INSTRUCTIONS

1. In a large bowl, combine chickpeas, cherry tomatoes, cucumber, red onion, olives, feta cheese, and parsley.
2. In a small bowl, whisk together olive oil, red wine vinegar, oregano, salt, and pepper.
3. Pour the dressing over the salad and toss to combine.
4. Serve immediately or refrigerate for up to 2 days to allow flavors to meld.

Nutritional Information (per serving):- Calories: 250- Protein: 8g- Carbohydrates: 24g- Fat: 14g- Fiber: 6g

10. BAKED SALMON WITH ASPARAGUS AND QUINOA

Servings: 04　　　**Prep. time:** 10 minutes　　　**Cook time:** 20 minutes

INGREDIENTS

- 4 salmon fillets (about 4 oz each)

- 1 tablespoon olive oil

- Salt and pepper to taste

- 1 teaspoon garlic powder

- 1 lemon, thinly sliced

- 1 lb asparagus, trimmed

- 1 cup quinoa, rinsed

- 2 cups water

- 2 tablespoons chopped fresh dill

INSTRUCTIONS

6. Preheat the oven to 400°F (200°C). Line a baking sheet with parchment paper.

7. Place the salmon fillets on the baking sheet. Drizzle with olive oil, and season with salt, pepper, and garlic powder. Top each fillet with a few lemon slices.

8. Arrange the asparagus around the salmon on the baking sheet, drizzle with a little olive oil, and season with salt and pepper.

9. Bake in the preheated oven for 12-15 minutes, or until the salmon is cooked through and flakes easily with a fork.

10. While the salmon is baking, bring 2 cups of water to a boil in a medium saucepan. Add quinoa, reduce heat to low, cover, and simmer for 15 minutes, or until the quinoa is tender and water is absorbed.

11. Serve the baked salmon and asparagus over a bed of quinoa, garnished with fresh dill.

Nutritional Information (per serving):- Calories: 380- Protein: 30g- Carbohydrates: 28g- Fat: 17g- Fiber: 5g

11. ZUCCHINI NOODLES WITH TOMATO SAUCE AND TURKEY MEATBALLS

Servings: 04   **Prep. time:** 10 minutes   **Cook time:** 20 minutes

INGREDIENTS

- 4 large zucchinis, spiralized
- 1 tablespoon olive oil
- 1 small onion, finely chopped
- 3 garlic cloves, minced
- 1 can (15 oz) crushed tomatoes
- 1 teaspoon dried oregano
- Salt and pepper to taste
- 1/2 cup fresh basil, chopped
- 1 lb ground turkey
- 1/4 cup whole wheat breadcrumbs
- 1 egg
- 1/4 cup grated Parmesan cheese

INSTRUCTIONS

1. In a large skillet, heat 1/2 tablespoon of olive oil over medium heat. Add the onion and garlic and cook for 5 minutes until softened.
2. Add the crushed tomatoes, oregano, salt, and pepper. Simmer for 15 minutes, stirring occasionally.
3. Meanwhile, in a bowl, mix the ground turkey, breadcrumbs, egg, Parmesan cheese, salt, and pepper. Form small meatballs.
4. In a separate skillet, heat the remaining 1/2 tablespoon of olive oil over medium-high heat and cook the meatballs for 7-8 minutes, turning until they are well browned and cooked through.
5. Add the meatballs to the tomato sauce and cook for another 5 minutes.
6. In the same skillet used for the meatballs, cook the zucchini noodles for 2-3 minutes until slightly tender.
7. Serve the zucchini noodles with the tomato sauce and turkey meatballs, garnished with fresh basil.

Nutritional Information (per serving):- Calories: 310- Protein: 28g- Carbohydrates: 18g- Fat: 15g- Fiber: 5g

12. BUDDHA BOWL WITH HUMMUS AND ROASTED VEGETABLES

Servings: 04

Prep. time: 20 minutes

Cook time: 30 minutes

INGREDIENTS

- 1 cup quinoa, rinsed

- 2 cups vegetable broth

- 1 cup canned chickpeas, drained and rinsed

- 1 tablespoon olive oil

- 1 teaspoon smoked paprika

- 1 medium sweet potato, diced

- 1 red bell pepper, sliced

- 1 cup kale, chopped

- 1 avocado, sliced

- 1/2 cup hummus

- 2 tablespoons toasted pumpkin seeds

- Juice of 1/2 lemon

- Salt and pepper to taste

INSTRUCTIONS

1. Preheat the oven to 400°F (200°C). Arrange the chickpeas, sweet potatoes, and bell pepper on a baking sheet, drizzle with olive oil, smoked paprika, salt, and pepper. Roast for 25-30 minutes, stirring halfway through, until golden and tender.

2. Meanwhile, bring the vegetable broth to a boil in a medium saucepan. Add the quinoa, reduce heat, cover, and simmer for 15 minutes, or until the quinoa is tender and the liquid is absorbed.

3. In a small skillet, heat a little olive oil and sauté the kale for 2-3 minutes until slightly wilted.

4. Divide the cooked quinoa into four bowls. Add the roasted chickpeas, sweet potatoes, bell peppers, sautéed kale, and sliced avocado.

5. Add a dollop of hummus to each bowl, sprinkle with toasted pumpkin seeds, and drizzle with lemon juice.

6. Serve immediately or store in the fridge for up to 3 days.

Nutritional Information (per serving):- Calories: 420- Protein: 12g- Carbohydrates: 52g- Fat: 18g- Fiber: 12g

13. WHOLE WHEAT BANANA NUT MUFFINS

Servings: 04   **Prep. time:** 20 minutes   **Cook time:** 30 minutes

INGREDIENTS

- 1 1/2 cups whole wheat flour
- 1/2 cup coconut sugar
- 1 teaspoon baking powder
- 1/2 teaspoon baking soda
- 1/2 teaspoon ground cinnamon
- 1/4 teaspoon salt
- 3 ripe bananas, mashed
- 1 large egg
- 1/4 cup melted coconut oil
- 1/4 cup unsweetened almond milk
- 1 teaspoon vanilla extract
- 1/2 cup chopped walnuts

INSTRUCTIONS

1. Preheat the oven to 350°F (175°C). Line a muffin tin with paper liners.
2. In a large bowl, mix together the whole wheat flour, coconut sugar, baking powder, baking soda, cinnamon, and salt.
3. In a separate bowl, combine the mashed bananas, egg, melted coconut oil, almond milk, and vanilla extract. Mix until smooth.
4. Add the wet ingredients to the dry ingredients and stir until just combined. Gently fold in the chopped walnuts.
5. Fill the muffin liners about 3/4 full. Bake in the preheated oven for 18-20 minutes, or until a toothpick inserted in the center comes out clean.
6. Let the muffins cool in the tin for 5 minutes before transferring them to a wire rack to cool completely.

Nutritional Information (per serving):- Calories: 180- Protein: 4g- Carbohydrates: 28g- Fat: 7g- Fiber: 3g

14. KALE, APPLE, AND PECAN SALAD WITH LEMON VINAIGRETTE

Servings: 04

Prep. time: 15 minutes

Cook time: 00 minutes

INGREDIENTS

- 6 cups kale, chopped, stems removed

- 1 Granny Smith apple, thinly sliced

- 1/2 cup toasted pecans

- 1/4 cup crumbled feta cheese

- 1/4 cup dried cranberries

- 2 tablespoons extra virgin olive oil

- Juice of 1 lemon

- 1 tablespoon maple syrup

- 1 teaspoon Dijon mustard

- Salt and pepper to taste

INSTRUCTIONS

1. In a large bowl, combine the chopped kale, sliced apple, toasted pecans, crumbled feta cheese, and dried cranberries.

2. In a small bowl, prepare the vinaigrette by mixing olive oil, lemon juice, maple syrup, Dijon mustard, salt, and pepper. Whisk well until all ingredients are well combined.

3. Pour the vinaigrette over the salad and massage the kale with your hands for 2-3 minutes, until it becomes more tender.

4. Serve immediately or refrigerate until ready to serve.

Nutritional Information (per serving):- Calories: 220- Protein: 5g- Carbohydrates: 22g- Fat: 14g- Fiber: 5g

Servings: 04   **Prep. time:** 15 minutes   **Cook time:** 30 minutes

INGREDIENTS

- 1 tablespoon coconut oil

- 1 large onion, chopped

- 3 garlic cloves, minced

- 1 tablespoon fresh ginger, grated

- 1 red bell pepper, sliced

- 1 medium zucchini, sliced into rounds

- 1 lb chicken breast, cubed

- 2 tablespoons red curry paste

- 1 can (14 oz) light coconut milk

- 1 cup low-sodium chicken broth

- 1 cup fresh or frozen peas

- Juice of 1 lime

- 1/4 cup fresh cilantro, chopped

INSTRUCTIONS

1. Heat the coconut oil in a large skillet over medium heat. Add the onion and cook for 5 minutes until softened.
2. Add the garlic and ginger and cook for another 2 minutes.
3. Add the red bell pepper and zucchini and cook for 5 minutes until the vegetables start to soften.
4. Add the cubed chicken and cook for 5-7 minutes until the chicken is browned and cooked through.
5. Stir in the curry paste and cook for 1 minute to release its flavor.
6. Pour in the coconut milk and chicken broth. Bring to a boil, then reduce the heat and simmer for 10 minutes.
7. Add the peas and cook for another 3-4 minutes.
8. Remove from heat, add lime juice, and stir in fresh cilantro.
9. Serve hot with brown rice or quinoa.

Nutritional Information (per serving):- Calories: 350- Protein: 28g- Carbohydrates: 18g- Fat: 18g- Fiber: 4g

16. CHIA SEED PORRIDGE WITH MANGO AND COCONUT

Servings: 02

Prep. time: 5 minutes (+ overnight soaking)

Cook time: 00 minutes

INGREDIENTS

- 1/4 cup chia seeds

- 1 cup unsweetened almond milk

- 1 tablespoon maple syrup

- 1/2 teaspoon vanilla extract

- 1/2 cup fresh mango, diced

- 2 tablespoons unsweetened shredded coconut

- 1 tablespoon toasted sliced almonds

INSTRUCTIONS

1. In a medium bowl, mix chia seeds, almond milk, maple syrup, and vanilla extract.
2. Cover and let it sit in the refrigerator for at least 4 hours or overnight until the chia seeds absorb the liquid and the mixture thickens.
3. When ready to serve, divide the chia pudding into two bowls.
4. Top with diced mango, shredded coconut, and toasted almonds.
5. Serve chilled.

Nutritional Information (per serving):- Calories: 250- Protein: 6g- Carbohydrates: 28g- Fat: 13g- Fiber: 11g

Servings: 04   **Prep. time:** 20 minutes   **Cook time:** 40 minutes

INGREDIENTS

- 4 large bell peppers, tops cut off and seeds removed

- 1 cup quinoa, rinsed

- 2 cups low-sodium vegetable broth

- 1 tablespoon olive oil

- 1 small onion, chopped

- 2 garlic cloves, minced

- 1 can (15 oz) black beans, drained and rinsed

- 1 cup corn kernels (fresh, frozen, or canned)

- 1 teaspoon ground cumin

- 1 teaspoon smoked paprika

- Salt and pepper to taste

- 1/2 cup shredded cheddar cheese (optional)

- 1/4 cup chopped fresh cilantro

- 1 lime, cut into wedges

INSTRUCTIONS

1. Preheat the oven to 375°F (190°C). Arrange the bell peppers upright in a baking dish.

2. In a medium saucepan, bring the vegetable broth to a boil. Add the quinoa, reduce heat, cover, and simmer for 15 minutes until the quinoa is tender and the liquid is absorbed.

3. While the quinoa cooks, heat olive oil in a large skillet over medium heat. Add the onion and cook for 5 minutes until softened. Add garlic and cook for another 2 minutes.

4. Add the black beans, corn, cumin, smoked paprika, salt, and pepper to the skillet. Cook for 5 minutes until heated through.

5. Stir the cooked quinoa into the skillet and mix well.

6. Stuff each bell pepper with the quinoa and black bean mixture. Top with cheddar cheese, if using.

7. Cover the baking dish with foil and bake for 30 minutes. Remove the foil and bake for an additional 10 minutes until the cheese is melted and bubbly.

8. Garnish with chopped cilantro and serve with lime wedges.

Nutritional Information (per serving):- Calories: 280- Protein: 10g- Carbohydrates: 45g- Fat: 7g- Fiber: 12g

Servings: 04   **Prep. time:** 15minutes   **Cook time:** 30 minutes

INGREDIENTS

- 1 tablespoon coconut oil

- 1 large onion, chopped

- 2 garlic cloves, minced

- 1 tablespoon fresh ginger, grated

- 2 medium sweet potatoes, peeled and diced

- 1 cup red lentils, rinsed

- 1 can (14 oz) diced tomatoes

- 1 can (14 oz) coconut milk

- 2 cups vegetable broth

- 1 tablespoon curry powder

- 1 teaspoon ground turmeric

- Salt and pepper to taste

- 2 cups baby spinach

- 1/4 cup fresh cilantro, chopped

INSTRUCTIONS

1. Heat coconut oil in a large pot over medium heat. Add the onion and cook for 5 minutes until softened. Add the garlic and ginger and cook for another 2 minutes.
2. Add the diced sweet potatoes, red lentils, diced tomatoes, coconut milk, vegetable broth, curry powder, turmeric, salt, and pepper. Stir well to combine.
3. Bring to a boil, then reduce the heat to low and simmer for 25-30 minutes until the sweet potatoes are tender and the lentils are cooked through.
4. Stir in the baby spinach and cook for another 2-3 minutes until wilted.
5. Serve hot, garnished with fresh cilantro, over brown rice or with naan bread.

Nutritional Information (per serving):- Calories:320- Protein: 12g- Carbohydrates: 50g- Fat: 11g- Fiber: 14g

19. GRILLED SALMON WITH AVOCADO SALSA

Servings: 04   **Prep. time:** 10 minutes   **Cook time:** 10 minutes

INGREDIENTS

- 4 salmon fillets (about 6 oz each)

- 1 tablespoon olive oil

- Salt and pepper to taste

- 1 teaspoon smoked paprika

- Juice of 1 lime

- 1 avocado, diced

- 1/2 red onion, finely chopped

- 1 jalapeño, seeded and finely chopped

- 1/4 cup fresh cilantro, chopped

- 1 tablespoon olive oil

- Juice of 1 lime

INSTRUCTIONS

1. Preheat the grill to medium-high heat. Rub the salmon fillets with olive oil, smoked paprika, salt, pepper, and lime juice.

2. Grill the salmon for 4-5 minutes per side or until the fish is cooked to your desired level of doneness.

3. While the salmon is grilling, prepare the avocado salsa. In a medium bowl, combine diced avocado, red onion, jalapeño, cilantro, olive oil, and lime juice. Mix gently to combine and season with salt and pepper to taste.

4. Serve the grilled salmon topped with avocado salsa. Enjoy with a side of quinoa or mixed greens.

Nutritional Information (per serving):- Calories: 380- Protein: 30g- Carbohydrates: 10g- Fat: 26g- Fiber: 5g

20. MEDITERRANEAN CHICKPEA SALAD

Servings: 04   **Prep. time:** 15 minutes   **Cook time:** 00 minutes

INGREDIENTS

- 1 can (15 oz) chickpeas, drained and rinsed

- 1 cup cherry tomatoes, halved

- 1 cucumber, diced

- 1/2 red onion, finely chopped

- 1/4 cup Kalamata olives, sliced

- 1/4 cup feta cheese, crumbled

- 1/4 cup fresh parsley, chopped

- 2 tablespoons extra virgin olive oil

- Juice of 1 lemon

- 1 teaspoon dried oregano

- Salt and pepper to taste

INSTRUCTIONS

1. In a large bowl, combine chickpeas, cherry tomatoes, cucumber, red onion, olives, feta cheese, and parsley.
2. In a small bowl, whisk together olive oil, lemon juice, dried oregano, salt, and pepper.
3. Pour the dressing over the salad and toss gently to combine.
4. Serve immediately or chill in the refrigerator for up to 2 hours before serving.

Nutritional Information (per serving):- Calories: 250- Protein: 8g- Carbohydrates: 30g- Fat: 12g- Fiber: 7g

21. SPAGHETTI SQUASH WITH SPINACH AND PINE NUTS

Servings: 04 **Prep. time:** 10 minutes **Cook time:** 45 minutes

INGREDIENTS

- 1 large spaghetti squash

- 1 tablespoon olive oil

- 2 garlic cloves, minced

- 4 cups fresh spinach

- 1/4 cup pine nuts, toasted

- 1/4 cup grated Parmesan cheese (optional)

- Salt and pepper to taste

INSTRUCTIONS

1. Preheat the oven to 400°F (200°C). Cut the spaghetti squash in half lengthwise and scoop out the seeds.

2. Place the squash halves cut-side down on a baking sheet and roast for 40-45 minutes, until the flesh is tender.

3. Using a fork, scrape the flesh of the squash to create "noodles" and transfer to a large bowl.

4. In a skillet, heat olive oil over medium heat. Add garlic and cook for 1 minute until fragrant.

5. Add spinach to the skillet and cook until wilted, about 2 minutes.

6. Toss the spinach and garlic mixture with the spaghetti squash noodles. Stir in toasted pine nuts and Parmesan cheese, if using. Season with salt and pepper to taste.

7. Serve warm.

Nutritional Information (per serving):- Calories: 220- Protein: 6g- Carbohydrates: 25g- Fat: 12g- Fiber: 5g

22. GREEK YOGURT AND BERRY PARFAIT

Servings: 04   **Prep. time:** 10 minutes   **Cook time:** 00minutes

INGREDIENTS

- 2 cups plain Greek yogurt (non-fat or low-fat)

- 1 tablespoon honey or maple syrup

- 1 teaspoon vanilla extract

- 1 cup mixed berries (strawberries, blueberries, raspberries)

- 1/4 cup granola

- 2 tablespoons chia seeds

INSTRUCTIONS

1. In a bowl, mix the Greek yogurt with honey (or maple syrup) and vanilla extract.

2. In serving glasses or bowls, layer the yogurt mixture with mixed berries.

3. Sprinkle granola and chia seeds on top of each layer.

4. Repeat the layers until the glasses are filled.

5. Serve immediately or chill in the refrigerator for up to 2 hours before serving.

Nutritional Information (per serving):- Calories: 280- Protein: 15g- Carbohydrates: 35g- Fat: 10g- Fiber: 6g

23. LENTIL AND VEGETABLE SOUP

Servings: 06   **Prep. time:** 15 minutes   **Cook time:** 35 minutes

INGREDIENTS

- 1 tablespoon olive oil

- 1 large onion, chopped

- 2 garlic cloves, minced

- 2 carrots, diced

- 2 celery stalks, diced

- 1 cup dried green or brown lentils, rinsed

- 1 can (14 oz) diced tomatoes

- 4 cups vegetable broth

- 1 teaspoon dried thyme

- 1 bay leaf

- 2 cups chopped kale or spinach

- Salt and pepper to taste

INSTRUCTIONS

1. Heat olive oil in a large pot over medium heat. Add the onion, garlic, carrots, and celery. Cook for 5 minutes until the vegetables start to soften.

2. Add the lentils, diced tomatoes, vegetable broth, thyme, and bay leaf. Bring to a boil.

3. Reduce heat to low, cover, and simmer for 30 minutes, or until lentils and vegetables are tender.

4. Stir in the chopped kale or spinach and cook for another 5 minutes until wilted.

5. Season with salt and pepper to taste. Serve hot.

Nutritional Information (per serving):- Calories: 220- Protein: 12g- Carbohydrates: 35g- Fat: 4g- Fiber: 10g

24. SWEET POTATO AND BLACK BEAN TACOS

Servings: 04   **Prep. time:** 15 minutes   **Cook time:** 30 minutes

INGREDIENTS

- 2 large sweet potatoes, peeled and diced

- 1 tablespoon olive oil

- 1 teaspoon ground cumin

- 1 teaspoon smoked paprika

- 1/2 teaspoon garlic powder

- Salt and pepper to taste

- 1 can (15 oz) black beans, drained and rinsed

- 8 small corn tortillas

- 1 cup shredded cabbage

- 1/4 cup chopped fresh cilantro

- 1 avocado, sliced

- Lime wedges, for serving

INSTRUCTIONS

1. Preheat the oven to 400°F (200°C). Toss the diced sweet potatoes with olive oil, cumin, smoked paprika, garlic powder, salt, and pepper. Spread on a baking sheet and roast for 25-30 minutes, or until tender and slightly crispy.

2. Warm the corn tortillas in a dry skillet or oven.

3. Heat the black beans in a small saucepan over medium heat until warmed through.

4. To assemble the tacos, layer roasted sweet potatoes, black beans, shredded cabbage, and avocado slices on each tortilla.

5. Garnish with chopped cilantro and serve with lime wedges.

Nutritional Information (per serving, 2 tacos):- Calories: 300- Protein: 10g- Carbohydrates: 45g- Fat: 12g- Fiber: 09g

25. BAKED CHICKEN AND VEGETABLE SHEET PAN DINNER

Servings: 04   **Prep. time:** 10 minutes   **Cook time:** 30 minutes

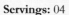

INGREDIENTS

- 4 bone-in, skinless chicken thighs

- 2 tablespoons olive oil

- 1 teaspoon garlic powder

- 1 teaspoon paprika

- 1/2 teaspoon dried thyme

- Salt and pepper to taste

- 2 cups baby carrots

- 1 cup broccoli florets

- 1 cup bell pepper, sliced

- 1 red onion, cut into wedges

INSTRUCTIONS

1. Preheat the oven to 425°F (220°C). Line a large baking sheet with parchment paper.
2. Rub the chicken thighs with olive oil, garlic powder, paprika, thyme, salt, and pepper.
3. Arrange the chicken thighs on the baking sheet and surround with carrots, broccoli, bell pepper, and red onion.
4. Roast in the oven for 25-30 minutes, or until the chicken reaches an internal temperature of 165°F (74°C) and the vegetables are tender.
5. Serve hot.

Nutritional Information (per serving, 1 chicken thigh with vegetables):- Calories: 350- Protein: 25g- Carbohydrates: 30g- Fat: 15g- Fiber: 08g

26. SPICY HUMMUS AND VEGGIE WRAPS

Servings: 04   **Prep. time:** 10 minutes   **Cook time:** 00 minutes

INGREDIENTS

- 1 cup spicy hummus (store-bought or homemade)

- 4 whole wheat tortillas

- 1 cup mixed greens

- 1 cup sliced bell peppers

- 1 cup shredded carrots

- 1/2 cucumber, sliced

- 1/4 cup red onion, thinly sliced

INSTRUCTIONS

1. Spread a generous layer of spicy hummus over each tortilla.
2. Layer mixed greens, bell peppers, shredded carrots, cucumber slices, and red onion on top of the hummus.
3. Roll up the tortillas tightly, then cut in half diagonally.
4. Serve immediately or wrap in foil for a portable lunch.

Nutritional Information (per wrap):- Calories: 250- Protein: 8g- Carbohydrates: 35g- Fat: 10g- Fiber: 08g

27. ALMOND-CRUSTED TILAPIA WITH STEAMED ASPARAGUS

Servings: 04   **Prep. time:** 10 minutes   **Cook time:** 20 minutes

INGREDIENTS

- 4 tilapia fillets (about 6 oz each)

- 1/2 cup almond meal

- 1/4 cup grated Parmesan cheese

- 1 egg, beaten

- Salt and pepper to taste

- 1 bunch asparagus, trimmed

- 1 tablespoon olive oil

- Juice of 1 lemon

INSTRUCTIONS

1. Preheat the oven to 375°F (190°C). Line a baking sheet with parchment paper.

2. In a shallow dish, combine almond meal, Parmesan cheese, salt, and pepper.

3. Dip each tilapia fillet in the beaten egg, then coat with the almond mixture. Place on the prepared baking sheet.

4. Bake for 15-20 minutes, or until the tilapia is cooked through and the coating is golden brown.

5. While the fish bakes, steam the asparagus until tender, about 5 minutes. Toss with olive oil and lemon juice.

6. Serve the almond-crusted tilapia with the steamed asparagus.

Nutritional Information (per wrap):- Calories: 320- Protein: 30g- Carbohydrates: 15g- Fat: 15g- Fiber: 05g

28. APPLE CINNAMON OVERNIGHT OATS

Servings: 01   **Prep. time:** 05 minutes   **Cook time:** 00 minutes

INGREDIENTS

- 1/2 cup rolled oats

- 1/2 cup unsweetened almond milk

- 1/2 cup plain Greek yogurt

- 1 apple, diced

- 1 tablespoon chia seeds

- 1 tablespoon maple syrup

- 1/2 teaspoon ground cinnamon

- 1/4 teaspoon vanilla extract

INSTRUCTIONS

1. In a jar or container, combine rolled oats, almond milk, Greek yogurt, chia seeds, maple syrup, cinnamon, and vanilla extract.
2. Stir well to combine and ensure the oats are fully submerged in the liquid.
3. Top with diced apple, cover, and refrigerate overnight.
4. In the morning, stir the oats and enjoy.

Nutritional Information (per serving):- Calories: 280- Protein: 14g- Carbohydrates: 40g- Fat: 8g- Fiber: 7g

Servings: 04   **Prep. time:** 10 minutes   **Cook time:** 25 minutes

INGREDIENTS

- 1 lb Brussels sprouts, trimmed and halved

- 2 tablespoons olive oil

- Salt and pepper to taste

- 2 tablespoons balsamic vinegar

- 1 tablespoon honey

- 1/4 cup toasted pine nuts

INSTRUCTIONS

1. Preheat the oven to 400°F (200°C). Line a baking sheet with parchment paper.

2. Toss the Brussels sprouts with olive oil, salt, and pepper. Spread them out in a single layer on the baking sheet.

3. Roast for 20-25 minutes, shaking the pan halfway through, until the Brussels sprouts are crispy on the outside and tender inside.

4. While the Brussels sprouts are roasting, prepare the balsamic glaze. In a small saucepan, combine balsamic vinegar and honey. Simmer over medium heat for 5-7 minutes, until reduced and thickened.

5. Drizzle the balsamic glaze over the roasted Brussels sprouts and sprinkle with toasted pine nuts.

6. Serve warm.

Nutritional Information (per serving):- Calories: 180- Protein: 4g- Carbohydrates: 20g- Fat: 10g- Fiber: 6g

30. ZUCCHINI NOODLES WITH PESTO AND CHERRY TOMATOES

Servings: 04   **Prep. time:** 10 minutes   **Cook time:** 10 minutes

INGREDIENTS

- 4 medium zucchinis, spiralized into noodles

- 1 cup cherry tomatoes, halved

- 1/4 cup pesto sauce (store-bought or homemade)

- 1 tablespoon olive oil

- Salt and pepper to taste

- 1/4 cup grated Parmesan cheese (optional)

INSTRUCTIONS

1. Heat olive oil in a large skillet over medium heat. Add the zucchini noodles and cook for 3-4 minutes, stirring occasionally, until slightly tender.

2. Add the cherry tomatoes and cook for another 2 minutes, until they start to soften.

3. Stir in the pesto sauce and cook for an additional 2 minutes, until everything is well coated and heated through.

4. Season with salt and pepper to taste. Serve with a sprinkle of Parmesan cheese, if desired.

Nutritional Information (per serving):- Calories: 150- Protein: 5g- Carbohydrates: 15g- Fat: 8g- Fiber: 4g

Servings: 01   **Prep. time:** 05 minutes   **Cook time:** 00 minutes

INGREDIENTS

- 1 banana, frozen

- 1/2 cup frozen berries (strawberries, blueberries, or raspberries)

- 1/2 cup plain Greek yogurt

- 1/2 cup unsweetened almond milk

- 1 tablespoon chia seeds

- 1 scoop protein powder (vanilla or unflavored)

- Toppings: freshfruit, granola, nuts, seeds,shredded coconut

INSTRUCTIONS

1. In a blender, combine the frozen banana, frozen berries, Greek yogurt, almond milk, chia seeds, and protein powder. Blend until smooth and creamy.

2. Pour the smoothie into a bowl and top with your choice of fresh fruit, granola, nuts, seeds, and shredded coconut.

3. Serve immediately.

Nutritional Information (per serving):- Calories: 300- Protein: 20g- Carbohydrates: 40g- Fat: 8g- Fiber: 7g

32. STUFFED PORTOBELLO MUSHROOMS

Servings: 04

Prep. time: 10 minutes

Cook time: 25 minutes

INGREDIENTS

- 4 large portobello mushrooms, stems removed

- 1 tablespoon olive oil

- 1 cup cooked quinoa

- 1/2 cup sun-dried tomatoes, chopped

- 1/2 cup spinach, chopped

- 1/4 cup feta cheese, crumbled

- 2 cloves garlic, minced

- 1/4 cup chopped fresh basil

- Salt and pepper to taste

INSTRUCTIONS

1. Preheat the oven to 375°F (190°C). Line a baking sheet with parchment paper.

2. Brush the portobello mushrooms with olive oil and place them on the baking sheet, gill side up.

3. In a bowl, combine the cooked quinoa, sun-dried tomatoes, spinach, feta cheese, garlic, basil, salt, and pepper.

4. Spoon the mixture evenly into the mushroom caps.

5. Bake for 20-25 minutes, until the mushrooms are tender and the filling is heated through.

6. Serve warm.

Nutritional Information (per serving):- Calories: 250- Protein: 10g- Carbohydrates: 30g- Fat: 10g- Fiber: 5g

33. CREAMY AVOCADO AND TOMATO SOUP

Servings: 04   **Prep. time:** 10 minutes   **Cook time:** 15 minutes

INGREDIENTS

- 2 ripe avocados, peeled and pitted

- 2 cups cherry tomatoes, halved

- 1/2 cup diced onion

- 2 garlic cloves, minced

- 2 cups vegetable broth

- 1 tablespoon olive oil

- 1/2 cup fresh basil leaves

- Salt and pepper to taste

INSTRUCTIONS

1. In a large pot, heat olive oil over medium heat. Add the diced onion and cook for 5 minutes, until softened.

2. Add the garlic and cook for another minute until fragrant.

3. Stir in the cherry tomatoes and cook for 5 minutes, until they start to break down.

4. Add the vegetable broth and bring to a boil. Reduce heat and simmer for 10 minutes.

5. Remove from heat and let cool slightly. Blend the soup with an immersion blender or in batches using a regular blender until smooth.

6. Return the soup to the pot and stir in the avocados and basil. Blend again until smooth and creamy.

7. Season with salt and pepper to taste. Serve hot or chilled.

Nutritional Information (per serving):- Calories: 220- Protein: 4g- Carbohydrates: 20g- Fat: 15g- Fiber: 7g

Servings: 04   **Prep. time:** 10 minutes   **Cook time:** 25 minutes

INGREDIENTS

- 12 large white mushrooms, stems removed

- 1 tablespoon olive oil

- 1/2 pound ground turkey

- 1 cup fresh spinach, chopped

- 1/4 cup onion, finely chopped

- 2 garlic cloves, minced

- 1/4 cup grated Parmesan cheese

- 1/4 cup whole wheat breadcrumbs

- Salt and pepper to taste

INSTRUCTIONS

1. Preheat the oven to 375°F (190°C). Line a baking sheet with parchment paper.

2. Heat olive oil in a skillet over medium heat. Add the onion and cook for 3-4 minutes until softened. Add garlic and cook for another minute.

3. Add ground turkey to the skillet and cook until browned, breaking it up with a spoon as it cooks.

4. Stir in the chopped spinach and cook for another 2 minutes until wilted. Remove from heat and let cool slightly.

5. In a bowl, combine the turkey mixture with Parmesan cheese and breadcrumbs. Season with salt and pepper.

6. Spoon the mixture into the mushroom caps and place them on the prepared baking sheet.

7. Bake for 15-20 minutes, until the mushrooms are tender and the tops are golden brown.

8. Serve warm.

Nutritional Information (per serving, 3 mushrooms):- Calories: 180- Protein: 15g- Carbohydrates: 10g- Fat: 10g- Fiber: 3g

35. CILANTRO LIME QUINOA SALAD

Servings: 04   **Prep. time:** 10 minutes   **Cook time:** 15 minutes

INGREDIENTS

- 1 cup quinoa, rinsed

- 2 cups water

- 1 cup cherry tomatoes, halved

- 1 cup corn kernels (fresh or frozen)

- 1/2 cup diced cucumber

- 1/4 cup red onion, finely chopped

- 1/4 cup fresh cilantro, chopped

- Juice of 2 limes

- 2 tablespoons olive oil

- Salt and pepper to taste

INSTRUCTIONS

1. In a medium saucepan, bring water to a boil. Add quinoa, reduce heat to low, cover, and simmer for 15 minutes or until the quinoa is cooked and the water is absorbed.

2. Let the quinoa cool slightly, then fluff with a fork and transfer to a large bowl.

3. Add cherry tomatoes, corn, cucumber, red onion, and cilantro to the quinoa.

4. In a small bowl, whisk together lime juice, olive oil, salt, and pepper.

5. Pour the dressing over the quinoa salad and toss to combine.

6. Serve chilled or at room temperature.

Nutritional Information (per serving):- Calories: 250- Protein: 8g- Carbohydrates: 35g- Fat: 10g- Fiber: 6g

36. CHICKEN AND VEGETABLE STIR-FRY

Servings: 04

Prep. time: 10 minutes

Cook time: 15 minutes

INGREDIENTS

- 1 tablespoon olive oil

- 1 lb boneless, skinless chicken breast, sliced into thin strips

- 2 cups broccoli florets

- 1 cup bell pepper, sliced

- 1 cup snap peas

- 2 garlic cloves, minced

- 1 tablespoon fresh ginger, grated

- 1/4 cup low-sodium soy sauce

- 2 tablespoons hoisin sauce

- 1 tablespoon rice vinegar

- 1 teaspoon sesame oil

- Cooked brown rice or quinoa, for serving

INSTRUCTIONS

1. Heat olive oil in a large skillet or wok over medium-high heat. Add chicken strips and cook until browned and cooked through, about 5-7 minutes. Remove from skillet and set aside.

2. In the same skillet, add broccoli, bell pepper, snap peas, garlic, and ginger. Stir-fry for 4-5 minutes, until the vegetables are tender-crisp.

3. Return the chicken to the skillet and add soy sauce, hoisin sauce, rice vinegar, and sesame oil. Stir to coat everything evenly and cook for another 2 minutes.

4. Serve the stir-fry over cooked brown rice or quinoa.

Nutritional Information (per serving with 1 cup brown rice):- Calories: 350- Protein: 30g- Carbohydrates: 45g- Fat: 10g- Fiber: 6g

37. BERRY CHIA JAM

Servings: 10　　　**Prep. time:** 10 minutes　　　**Cook time:** 10 minutes

INGREDIENTS

- 2 cups mixed berries (strawberries, blueberries, raspberries)

- 2 tablespoons honey or maple syrup

- 2 tablespoons chia seeds

- 1 teaspoon lemon juice

INSTRUCTIONS

1. In a medium saucepan, combine the mixed berries and honey. Cook over medium heat for 5-7 minutes, until the berries break down and the mixture starts to thicken.

2. Remove from heat and stir in chia seeds and lemon juice. Let the mixture cool slightly, then transfer to a jar.

3. Refrigerate for at least 2 hours to allow the chia seeds to thicken the jam.

4. Serve on toast, yogurt, or as a topping for oatmeal.

Nutritional Information (per tablespoon):- Calories: 30- Protein: 1g- Carbohydrates: 8g- Fat: 0g- Fiber: 2g

Servings: 04   **Prep. time:** 15 minutes   **Cook time:** 30 minutes

INGREDIENTS

- 1 tablespoon coconut oil

- 1 onion, chopped

- 2 garlic cloves, minced

- 1 tablespoon fresh ginger, grated

- 1 eggplant, diced

- 1 can (15 oz) chickpeas, drained and rinsed

- 1 can (14 oz) diced tomatoes

- 1 cup coconut milk

- 1 tablespoon curry powder

- 1 teaspoon ground turmeric

- 1/2 teaspoon ground cumin

- Salt and pepper to taste

- Cooked basmati rice, for serving

INSTRUCTIONS

1. Heat coconut oil in a large pot over medium heat. Add the onion and cook until softened, about 5 minutes. Add garlic and ginger and cook for another minute.

2. Add the diced eggplant and cook for 5-7 minutes, until slightly softened.

3. Stir in chickpeas, diced tomatoes, coconut milk, curry powder, turmeric, cumin, salt, and pepper. Bring to a simmer.

4. Reduce heat and cook for 20 minutes, until the eggplant is tender and the flavors have melded together.

5. Serve the curry over cooked basmati rice.

Nutritional Information (per serving with 1 cup rice):- Calories: 350- Protein: 10g- Carbohydrates: 45g- Fat: 15g- Fiber: 8g

Servings: 04   **Prep. time:** 10 minutes   **Cook time:** 00 minutes

INGREDIENTS

- 2 cups cooked chicken breast, shredded

- 1/2 cup plain Greek yogurt

- 1/4 cup mayonnaise (optional)

- 1 tablespoon Dijon mustard

- 1 celery stalk, diced

- 1/4 cup red grapes, halved

- 1/4 cup walnuts, chopped

- 1 tablespoon fresh parsley, chopped

- Salt and pepper to taste

INSTRUCTIONS

1. In a large bowl, combine Greek yogurt, mayonnaise (if using), Dijon mustard, salt, and pepper.

2. Add shredded chicken, celery, grapes, walnuts, and parsley. Mix until well combined.

3. Serve immediately or refrigerate for 1 hour to allow the flavors to meld.

4. Enjoy on its own, or with whole grain crackers or in a whole wheat wrap.

Nutritional Information (per serving, 1/2 cup):- Calories: 200- Protein: 20g- Carbohydrates: 10g- Fat: 10g- Fiber: 2g

Servings: 04   **Prep. time:** 15 minutes   **Cook time:** 25 minutes

INGREDIENTS

- 1 can (15 oz) chickpeas, drained and rinsed

- 1/2 cup fresh parsley, chopped

- 1/2 cup fresh cilantro, chopped

- 1 small onion, chopped

- 3 garlic cloves

- 1 teaspoon ground cumin

- 1 teaspoon ground coriander

- 1/2 teaspoon baking powder

- 1/4 cup whole wheat flour

- Salt and pepper to taste

- 2 tablespoons olive oil

For the Tahini Sauce:

- 1/4 cup tahini

- Juice of 1 lemon

- 1 garlic clove, minced

- 2-3 tablespoons water (to thin)

INSTRUCTIONS

1. In a large bowl, combine Greek yogurt, mayonnaise (if using), Dijon mustard, salt, and pepper.
2. Add shredded chicken, celery, grapes, walnuts, and parsley. Mix until well combined.
3. Serve immediately or refrigerate for 1 hour to allow the flavors to meld.
4. Enjoy on its own, or with whole grain crackers or in a whole wheat wrap.

Nutritional Information (per serving, 4 falafel balls with 2 tablespoons sauce):- Calories: 250- Protein: 10g- Carbohydrates: 30g- Fat: 12g- Fiber: 8g

41. SPAGHETTI SQUASH WITH MARINARA SAUCE

Servings: 04　　　**Prep. time:** 10 minutes　　　**Cook time:** 45 minutes

INGREDIENTS

- 1 medium spaghetti squash

- 2 tablespoons olive oil

- 2 cups marinara sauce (store-bought or homemade)

- 1/4 cup grated Parmesan cheese

- Fresh basil leaves for garnish

- Salt and pepper to taste

INSTRUCTIONS

1. Preheat the oven to 400°F (200°C). Cut the spaghetti squash in half lengthwise and remove seeds.

2. Brush the cut sides with olive oil and season with salt and pepper. Place cut side down on a baking sheet.

3. Roast for 40-45 minutes, until tender. Let cool slightly.

4. Use a fork to scrape the flesh into spaghetti-like strands.

5. Heat marinara sauce in a saucepan over medium heat.

6. Toss the spaghetti squash with marinara sauce. Serve topped with Parmesan cheese and fresh basil.

Nutritional Information (per serving, 1 cup squash with 1/2 cup sauce):- Calories: 150- Protein: 6g- Carbohydrates: 20g- Fat: 6g- Fiber: 5g

42. ALMOND BUTTER ENERGY BALLS

Servings: 12   **Prep. time:** 10 minutes   **Cook time:** 30 minutes

INGREDIENTS

- 1 cup rolled oats

- 1/2 cup almond butter

- 1/4 cup honey or maple syrup

- 1/4 cup chia seeds

- 1/4 cup dark chocolate chips (optional)

- 1/4 cup shredded coconut (optional)

INSTRUCTIONS

1. In a large bowl, combine oats, almond butter, honey, chia seeds, and chocolate chips.
2. Mix until well combined. If the mixture is too dry, add a little more almond butter or honey.
3. Roll the mixture into 1-inch balls and place on a parchment-lined baking sheet.
4. Refrigerate for at least 30 minutes to firm up.
5. Store in an airtight container in the refrigerator for up to 1 week.

Nutritional Information (per serving, 1 ball):- Calories: 100- Protein: 3g- Carbohydrates: 12g- Fat: 5g- Fiber: 3g

43. ROASTED SWEET POTATO AND BLACK BEAN SALAD

Servings: 12

Prep. time: 10 minutes

Cook time: 25 minutes

INGREDIENTS

- 2 medium sweet potatoes, peeled and diced

- 1 tablespoon olive oil

- 1/2 teaspoon ground cumin

- 1/2 teaspoon smoked paprika

- Salt and pepper to taste

- 1 can (15 oz) black beans, drained and rinsed

- 1/4 cup red onion, finely chopped

- 1/4 cup fresh cilantro, chopped

- Juice of 1 lime

- 2 tablespoons olive oil

INSTRUCTIONS

1. Preheat the oven to 425°F (220°C). Line a baking sheet with parchment paper.
2. Toss the sweet potatoes with olive oil, cumin, paprika, salt, and pepper. Spread in a single layer on the baking sheet.
3. Roast for 20-25 minutes, until tender and slightly crispy.
4. In a large bowl, combine roasted sweet potatoes, black beans, red onion, and cilantro.
5. In a small bowl, whisk together lime juice and olive oil. Pour over the salad and toss to combine.
6. Serve warm or at room temperature.

Nutritional Information (per serving):- Calories: 250- Protein: 8g- Carbohydrates: 40g- Fat: 8g- Fiber: 10g

44. LENTIL AND VEGETABLE STEW

Servings: 06   **Prep. time:** 10 minutes   **Cook time:** 35 minutes

INGREDIENTS

- 1 tablespoon olive oil

- 1 onion, chopped

- 2 garlic cloves, minced

- 2 carrots, diced

- 2 celery stalks, diced

- 1 bell pepper, diced

- 1 cup dried green or brown lentils, rinsed

- 1 can (14.5 oz) diced tomatoes

- 4 cups vegetable broth

- 1 teaspoon dried thyme

- 1 teaspoon dried oregano

- Salt and pepper to taste

- 2 cups kale or spinach, chopped

INSTRUCTIONS

1. Heat olive oil in a large pot over medium heat. Add onion and cook until softened, about 5 minutes. Add garlic and cook for another minute.

2. Add carrots, celery, and bell pepper. Cook for 5-7 minutes, until vegetables begin to soften.

3. Stir in lentils, diced tomatoes, vegetable broth, thyme, oregano, salt, and pepper.

4. Bring to a boil, then reduce heat to low. Simmer for 25-30 minutes, until lentils are tender.

5. Stir in chopped kale or spinach and cook for another 5 minutes, until greens are wilted.

6. Serve hot.

Nutritional Information (per serving, 1 cup):- Calories: 200- Protein: 12g- Carbohydrates: 35g- Fat: 3g- Fiber: 10g

Servings: 04   **Prep. time:** 10 minutes   **Cook time:** 00 minutes

INGREDIENTS

- 1 ripe mango, peeled and diced

- 1 can (15 oz) black beans, drained and rinsed

- 1 red bell pepper, diced

- 1/4 cup red onion, finely chopped

- 1/4 cup fresh cilantro, chopped

- Juice of 1 lime

- Salt and pepper to taste

INSTRUCTIONS

1. In a large bowl, combine mango, black beans, red bell pepper, red onion, and cilantro.

2. Drizzle with lime juice and season with salt and pepper. Toss to combine.

3. Serve immediately with tortilla chips or as a topping for grilled chicken or fish.

Nutritional Information (per serving, 1 ball):- Calories: 150- Protein: 6g- Carbohydrates: 25g- Fat: 1g- Fiber: 6g

46. SWEET POTATO AND KALE FRITTATA

Servings: 06   **Prep. time:** 10 minutes   **Cook time:** 20 minutes

INGREDIENTS

- 1 tablespoon olive oil

- 1 medium sweet potato, peeled and diced

- 1/2 cup onion, chopped

- 2 cups kale, chopped

- 6 large eggs

- 1/4 cup milk (dairy or non-dairy)

- 1/2 cup shredded cheddar cheese (optional)

- Salt and pepper to taste

INSTRUCTIONS

1. Preheat the oven to 375°F (190°C). Heat olive oil in an oven-safe skillet over medium heat.

2. Add sweet potato and onion. Cook, stirring occasionally, for 10 minutes until sweet potato is tender.

3. Stir in kale and cook for another 2 minutes until wilted.

4. In a bowl, whisk together eggs, milk, salt, and pepper. Pour over the sweet potato mixture in the skillet.

5. Sprinkle cheese on top, if using.

6. Transfer the skillet to the oven and bake for 15-20 minutes, until the frittata is set and lightly browned.

7. Let cool slightly before slicing.

Nutritional Information (per serving, 1/6 of frittata):- Calories: 220- Protein: 14g- Carbohydrates: 20g- Fat: 12g- Fiber: 4g

Servings: 04   **Prep. time:** 15 minutes   **Cook time:** 30 minutes

INGREDIENTS

- 4 large bell peppers (any color)

- 1 cup cooked quinoa

- 1 can (15 oz) black beans, drained and rinsed

- 1 cup corn kernels (fresh or frozen)

- 1/2 cup diced tomatoes

- 1/4 cup chopped fresh cilantro

- 1 teaspoon cumin

- 1/2 teaspoon smoked paprika

- Salt and pepper to taste

- 1/2 cup shredded cheese (optional)

INSTRUCTIONS

1. Preheat the oven to 375°F (190°C). Cut the tops off the bell peppers and remove the seeds and membranes.

2. In a large bowl, combine cooked quinoa, black beans, corn, diced tomatoes, cilantro, cumin, paprika, salt, and pepper.

3. Stuff each bell pepper with the quinoa mixture and place them upright in a baking dish.

4. Top with shredded cheese, if using.

5. Bake for 25-30 minutes, until the peppers are tender and the cheese is melted.

6. Serve warm.

Nutritional Information (per stuffed pepper):- Calories: 250- Protein: 12g- Carbohydrates: 35g- Fat: 8g- Fiber: 8g

48. ALMOND-CRUSTED SALMON

 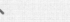

Servings: 04   **Prep. time:** 10 minutes   **Cook time:** 20 minutes

INGREDIENTS

- 4 salmon fillets

- 1/2 cup almond meal

- 1/4 cup grated Parmesan cheese

- 1 teaspoon dried thyme

- 1 teaspoon dried rosemary

- 1 tablespoon olive oil

- Salt and pepper to taste

INSTRUCTIONS

1. Preheat the oven to 400°F (200°C). Line a baking sheet with parchment paper.

2. In a shallow dish, combine almond meal, Parmesan cheese, thyme, rosemary, salt, and pepper.

3. Brush each salmon fillet with olive oil, then press into the almond mixture to coat.

4. Place the coated salmon fillets on the prepared baking sheet.

5. Bake for 15-20 minutes, until the salmon is cooked through and the crust is golden brown.

6. Serve with a side of steamed vegetables or a fresh salad.

Nutritional Information (per serving, 1 fillet):- Calories: 300- Protein: 25g- Carbohydrates: 8g- Fat: 20g- Fiber: 2g

49. CAULIFLOWER FRIED RICE

Servings: 04   **Prep. time:** 10 minutes   **Cook time:** 15 minutes

INGREDIENTS

- 1 large head of cauliflower, grated or processed into rice-sized pieces

- 2 tablespoons sesame oil

- 1/2 cup onion, chopped

- 2 garlic cloves, minced

- 1 cup mixed vegetables (carrots, peas, corn)

- 2 large eggs, beaten

- 3 tablespoons low-sodium soy sauce

- 1 green onion, sliced

- Salt and pepper to taste

INSTRUCTIONS

1. Heat sesame oil in a large skillet or wok over medium-high heat. Add onion and cook until softened, about 3 minutes. Add garlic and cook for another minute.

2. Add mixed vegetables and cook for 5 minutes until tender.

3. Push vegetables to one side of the skillet. Pour beaten eggs into the empty side and scramble until cooked through.

4. Add cauliflower rice and soy sauce to the skillet. Stir to combine and cook for 5-7 minutes until the cauliflower is tender and slightly golden.

5. Garnish with green onion and season with salt and pepper. Serve warm.

Nutritional Information (per serving, 1 cup):- Calories: 150- Protein: 7g- Carbohydrates: 15g- Fat: 8g- Fiber: 5g

Servings: 04   **Prep. time:** 10 minutes   **Cook time:** 07 minutes

INGREDIENTS

- 1 can (15 oz) chickpeas, drained and rinsed

- 1 tablespoon olive oil

- 1 teaspoon smoked paprika

- 1/2 teaspoon ground cumin

- 1/4 teaspoon cayenne pepper

- Salt to taste

- 1 ripe avocado, sliced

- 1/2 cup diced tomatoes

- 1/4 cup chopped fresh cilantro

- 4 whole wheat tortillas

INSTRUCTIONS

1. Heat olive oil in a skillet over medium heat. Add chickpeas, smoked paprika, cumin, cayenne pepper, and salt. Cook, stirring occasionally, for 5-7 minutes until chickpeas are crispy.

2. Warm tortillas in a dry skillet or microwave.

3. Spread chickpeas in the center of each tortilla. Top with avocado slices, diced tomatoes, and cilantro.

4. Roll up the tortillas, folding in the sides to create a wrap.

5. Serve immediately or wrap in foil for a portable lunch.

Nutritional Information (per wrap):- Calories: 300- Protein: 10g- Carbohydrates: 35g- Fat: 15g- Fiber: 8g

Servings: 04   **Prep. time:** 10 minutes   **Cook time:** 00 minutes

INGREDIENTS

- 4 medium zucchinis, spiralized into noodles

- 1/4 cup olive oil

- 1/2 cup basil leaves

- 1/4 cup pine nuts

- 1/4 cup grated Parmesan cheese

- 2 garlic cloves

- Juice of 1 lemon

- Salt and pepper to taste

INSTRUCTIONS

1. In a food processor, combine basil, pine nuts, Parmesan cheese, garlic, and lemon juice. Pulse until finely chopped.

2. With the food processor running, slowly drizzle in olive oil until the pesto is smooth. Season with salt and pepper.

3. Toss zucchini noodles with pesto until well coated.

4. Serve immediately, or lightly sauté the noodles in a skillet for 2-3 minutes for a warm dish.

Nutritional Information (per serving, 1 cup):- Calories: 200- Protein: 6g- Carbohydrates: 15g- Fat: 15g- Fiber: 4g

52. BAKED APPLE CHIPS

Servings: 04   **Prep. time:** 10 minutes   **Cook time:** 02 hours

INGREDIENTS

- 4 large apples, cored and thinly sliced

- 1 teaspoon ground cinnamon

- 1/4 teaspoon ground nutmeg

INSTRUCTIONS

1. Preheat the oven to 225°F (110°C). Line a baking sheet with parchment paper.
2. Arrange apple slices in a single layer on the baking sheet.
3. Sprinkle cinnamon and nutmeg evenly over the apple slices.
4. Bake for 1.5 to 2 hours, turning the slices halfway through, until they are crisp and dry.
5. Allow to cool before serving. Store in an airtight container.

Nutritional Information (per serving, 10 apple chips):- Calories: 70- Protein: 0g- Carbohydrates: 19g- Fat: 0g- Fiber: 3g

53. GREEK YOGURT AND BERRY PARFAIT

Servings: 04   **Prep. time:** 10 minutes   **Cook time:** 00 minutes

INGREDIENTS

- 2 cups plain Greek yogurt

- 1 cup mixed berries (strawberries, blueberries, raspberries)

- 1/4 cup granola

- 2 tablespoons honey or maple syrup

- Fresh mint leaves for garnish (optional

INSTRUCTIONS

1. In serving glasses or bowls, layer Greek yogurt with mixed berries and granola.
2. Drizzle with honey or maple syrup.
3. Garnish with fresh mint leaves if desired.
4. Serve immediately or refrigerate for up to 2 hours.

Nutritional Information (per serving, 1 parfait):- Calories: 250- Protein: 15g- Carbohydrates: 35g- Fat: 8g- Fiber: 5g

54. TURMERIC ROASTED CAULIFLOWER

Servings: 04

Prep. time: 10 minutes

Cook time: 30 minutes

INGREDIENTS

- 1 large head of cauliflower, cut into florets

- 2 tablespoons olive oil

- 1 teaspoon ground turmeric

- 1/2 teaspoon ground cumin

- 1/2 teaspoon smoked paprika

- Salt and pepper to taste

- 1 tablespoon lemon juice

- 1/4 cup fresh parsley, chopped

INSTRUCTIONS

1. Preheat the oven to 425°F (220°C). Line a baking sheet with parchment paper.

2. In a large bowl, toss cauliflower florets with olive oil, turmeric, cumin, smoked paprika, salt, and pepper.

3. Spread the cauliflower in a single layer on the prepared baking sheet.

4. Roast for 25-30 minutes, until golden and tender, tossing halfway through cooking.

5. Drizzle with lemon juice and garnish with fresh parsley before serving.

Nutritional Information (per serving, 1 cup):- Calories: 100- Protein: 3g- Carbohydrates: 10g- Fat: 7g- Fiber: 3g

Servings: 04   **Prep. time:** 15 minutes   **Cook time:** 00 minutes

INGREDIENTS

- 1 cup quinoa, rinsed and cooked

- 1/2 cup cherry tomatoes, halved

- 1/2 cup cucumber, diced

- 1/4 cup Kalamata olives, sliced

- 1/4 cup red onion, thinly sliced

- 1/4 cup feta cheese, crumbled

- 2 tablespoons fresh parsley, chopped

- 2 tablespoons olive oil

- 1 tablespoon red wine vinegar

- Salt and pepper to taste

INSTRUCTIONS

1. In a large bowl, combine cooked quinoa, cherry tomatoes, cucumber, olives, red onion, feta cheese, and parsley.

2. In a small bowl, whisk together olive oil, red wine vinegar, salt, and pepper.

3. Drizzle the dressing over the quinoa mixture and toss to combine.

4. Serve chilled or at room temperature.

Nutritional Information (per serving, 1 bowl):- Calories:250- Protein: 8g- Carbohydrates: 25g- Fat: 14g- Fiber: 4g

Servings: 04   **Prep. time:** 10 minutes   **Cook time:** 15 minutes

INGREDIENTS

- 8 oz whole wheat spaghetti

- 1/4 cup extra virgin olive oil

- 4 garlic cloves, thinly sliced

- 1/4 teaspoon red pepper flakes

- 4 cups fresh spinach, roughly chopped

- 1/4 cup grated Parmesan cheese

- Salt and pepper to taste

- Juice of 1/2 lemon

INSTRUCTIONS

1. Cook spaghetti according to package instructions until al dente. Reserve 1/2 cup of pasta water and drain the rest.

2. In a large skillet, heat olive oil over medium heat. Add garlic and red pepper flakes. Cook for 1-2 minutes until garlic is fragrant and lightly golden.

3. Add spinach to the skillet and cook for 2-3 minutes until wilted.

4. Add cooked spaghetti to the skillet and toss to coat in the garlic oil. Add reserved pasta water if needed to thin the sauce.

5. Remove from heat and stir in Parmesan cheese, salt, pepper, and lemon juice.

6. Serve immediately, garnished with extra Parmesan if desired.

Nutritional Information (per serving, 1 cup):- Calories:350- Protein: 12g- Carbohydrates: 45g- Fat: 15g- Fiber: 7g

57. AVOCADO CHOCOLATE MOUSSE

Servings: 04   **Prep. time:** 10 minutes   **Cook time:** 30 minutes

INGREDIENTS

- 2 ripe avocados

- 1/4 cup unsweetened cocoa powder

- 1/4 cup maple syrup or honey

- 1/4 cup almond milk

- 1 teaspoon vanilla extract

- A pinch of salt

- Fresh berries for topping (optional)

INSTRUCTIONS

1. In a food processor, blend avocados, cocoa powder, maple syrup, almond milk, vanilla extract, and salt until smooth and creamy.
2. Taste and adjust sweetness if needed by adding more maple syrup.
3. Divide the mousse into serving bowls and chill for at least 30 minutes before serving.
4. Top with fresh berries, if desired.

Nutritional Information (per serving, 1/2 cup):- Calories:200- Protein: 3g- Carbohydrates: 24g- Fat: 12g- Fiber: 7g

58. LEMON HERB GRILLED CHICKEN

Servings: 04   **Prep. time:** 10 minutes   **Marinate Time:** 30 minutes   **Cook time:** 12 minutes

INGREDIENTS

- 4 boneless, skinless chicken breasts

- 1/4 cup olive oil

- 2 tablespoons lemon juice

- 2 tablespoons fresh parsley, chopped

- 2 garlic cloves, minced

- 1 teaspoon dried oregano

- Salt and pepper to taste

INSTRUCTIONS

1. In a small bowl, whisk together olive oil, lemon juice, parsley, garlic, oregano, salt, and pepper.

2. Place chicken breasts in a large resealable bag and pour in the marinade. Seal the bag and refrigerate for at least 30 minutes, or up to 4 hours.

3. Preheat the grill to medium-high heat. Grill chicken for 5-6 minutes on each side, or until fully cooked and juices run clear.

4. Let the chicken rest for 5 minutes before serving. Serve with a side salad or steamed vegetables.

Nutritional Information (per serving, 1 chicken breast):- Calories:250- Protein: 30g- Carbohydrates: 2g- Fat: 12g- Fiber: 0g

59. COCONUT CHIA PUDDING

Servings: 04   **Prep. time:** 05 minutes   **Chill time:** 4 hours

INGREDIENTS

- 1/4 cup chia seeds

- 1 cup coconut milk

- 1 tablespoon maple syrup or honey

- 1/2 teaspoon vanilla extract

- Fresh fruit (berries, mango, kiwi) for topping

INSTRUCTIONS

1. In a medium bowl, whisk together chia seeds, coconut milk, maple syrup, and vanilla extract.

2. Cover and refrigerate for at least 4 hours or overnight until the chia seeds have absorbed the liquid and the pudding is thickened.

3. Stir the pudding before serving and divide it into bowls. Top with fresh fruit.

Nutritional Information (per serving, 1/2 cup):- Calories:180- Protein: 4g- Carbohydrates: 12g- Fat: 14g- Fiber: 8g

60. SWEET POTATO AND BLACK BEAN TACOS

Servings: 4 (8 tacos)   **Prep. time:** 10 minutes   **Chill time:** 25 minutes

INGREDIENTS

- 2 medium sweet potatoes, peeled and diced

- 2 tablespoons olive oil

- 1 teaspoon ground cumin

- 1/2 teaspoon smoked paprika

- Salt and pepper to taste

- 1 can (15 oz) black beans, drained and rinsed

- 8 small corn tortillas

- 1/2 cup red cabbage, thinly sliced

- 1/4 cup crumbled feta cheese (optional)

- 1/4 cup fresh cilantro, chopped

- 1 lime, cut into wedges

INSTRUCTIONS

1. Preheat the oven to 400°F (200°C). Toss diced sweet potatoes with olive oil, cumin, smoked paprika, salt, and pepper. Spread on a baking sheet and roast for 20-25 minutes, until tender and slightly crispy.

2. While sweet potatoes are roasting, warm the black beans in a small saucepan over medium heat.

3. Warm tortillas in a dry skillet or in the oven for a few minutes.

4. Assemble tacos by layering roasted sweet potatoes, black beans, red cabbage, and feta cheese on each tortilla.

5. Garnish with cilantro and serve with lime wedges.

Nutritional Information (per taco):- Calories:150- Protein: 5g- Carbohydrates: 25g- Fat:4g- Fiber: 6g

61. BERRY AND SPINACH SMOOTHIE BOWL

Servings: 01   **Prep. time:** 05 minutes   **Cook time:** 00 minutes

INGREDIENTS

- 1 cup frozen mixed berries

- 1/2 banana

- 1 cup fresh spinach

- 1/2 cup unsweetened almond milk

- 1 tablespoon chia seeds

- 1 tablespoon almond butter

- Granola, fresh fruit, and nuts for topping

INSTRUCTIONS

1. In a blender, combine frozen berries, banana, spinach, almond milk, chia seeds, and almond butter. Blend until smooth and thick.

2. Pour the smoothie into a bowl and top with granola, fresh fruit, and nuts.

3. Serve immediately.

Nutritional Information (per bowl):- Calories:250- Protein: 6g- Carbohydrates: 40g- Fat:8g- Fiber: 10g

Servings: 04   **Prep. time:** 10 minutes   **Cook time:** 15 minutes

INGREDIENTS

- 4 cod fillets

- 1/2 cup whole wheat breadcrumbs

- 1/4 cup Parmesan cheese, grated

- 1 tablespoon fresh parsley, chopped

- 1 tablespoon fresh dill, chopped

- 1 tablespoon olive oil

- 1 lemon, zested and juiced

- Salt and pepper to taste

INSTRUCTIONS

1. Preheat the oven to 375°F (190°C). Line a baking sheet with parchment paper.

2. In a small bowl, mix breadcrumbs, Parmesan cheese, parsley, dill, olive oil, lemon zest, salt, and pepper.

3. Pat cod fillets dry with a paper towel and place them on the prepared baking sheet. Spread the breadcrumb mixture evenly over the top of each fillet.

4. Bake for 12-15 minutes, until the fish is cooked through and the crust is golden.

5. Drizzle with lemon juice and serve with a side of steamed vegetables or a salad.

Nutritional Information (per fillet):- Calories:220- Protein: 30g- Carbohydrates: 8g- Fat: 8g- Fiber: 1g

Servings: 04   **Prep. time:** 10 minutes   **Cook time:** 20 minutes

INGREDIENTS

- 4 large Portobello mushrooms, stems removed

- 1 tablespoon olive oil

- 1 small onion, diced

- 2 garlic cloves, minced

- 1 cup spinach, chopped

- 1/2 cup cherry tomatoes, halved

- 1/4 cup walnuts, chopped

- 1/4 cup nutritional yeast

- Salt and pepper to taste

INSTRUCTIONS

1. Preheat the oven to 375°F (190°C). Line a baking sheet with parchment paper.

2. Brush Portobello mushrooms with olive oil and place them on the prepared baking sheet, gill side up.

3. In a skillet over medium heat, sauté onion and garlic in olive oil for 3-4 minutes, until softened. Add spinach, cherry tomatoes, walnuts, nutritional yeast, salt, and pepper. Cook for 2-3 minutes until spinach is wilted.

4. Spoon the mixture into the mushroom caps.

5. Bake for 15-20 minutes, until the mushrooms are tender.

6. Serve hot as a main dish or side.

Nutritional Information (per mushroom):- Calories:180- Protein: 6g- Carbohydrates: 14g- Fat: 12g- Fiber: 5g

Servings: 04   **Prep. time:** 15 minutes   **Cook time:** 00 minutes

INGREDIENTS

- 2 cups shredded rotisserie chicken

- 4 cups shredded cabbage (green or purple)

- 1 cup shredded carrots

- 1/2 cup red bell pepper, thinly sliced

- 1/4 cup chopped green onions

- 1/4 cup cilantro, chopped

- 1/4 cup chopped peanuts

FOR THE DRESSING

- 1/4 cup peanut butter

- 2 tablespoons rice vinegar

- 1 tablespoon soy sauce

- 1 tablespoon honey or maple syrup

- 1 tablespoon sesame oil

- 1 teaspoon grated ginger

- Juice of 1 lime

INSTRUCTIONS

1. In a large bowl, combine chicken, cabbage, carrots, bell pepper, green onions, and cilantro.

2. In a small bowl, whisk together peanut butter, rice vinegar, soy sauce, honey, sesame oil, ginger, and lime juice until smooth.

3. Pour the dressing over the salad and toss to combine.

4. Top with chopped peanuts before serving.

Nutritional Information (per serving, 1 cup):- Calories:300- Protein: 18g- Carbohydrates: 18g- Fat: 18g- Fiber: 5g

Servings: 04   **Prep. time:** 03 minutes   **Chill time:** 05 minutes

INGREDIENTS

- 4 medium zucchinis, spiralized

- 1 ripe avocado

- 1/4 cup fresh basil leaves

- 1/4 cup pine nuts

- 1/4 cup Parmesan cheese, grated

- 2 tablespoons olive oil

- 1 garlic clove, minced

- Juice of 1 lemon

- Salt and pepper to taste

- Cherry tomatoes, halved (optional)

INSTRUCTIONS

1. In a food processor, combine avocado, basil, pine nuts, Parmesan cheese, olive oil, garlic, lemon juice, salt, and pepper. Blend until smooth and creamy.

2. Heat a large skillet over medium heat. Add zucchini noodles and sauté for 2-3 minutes until slightly softened.

3. Remove from heat and toss the zucchini noodles with the avocado pesto until well coated.

4. Top with cherry tomatoes, if desired, and serve immediately.

Nutritional Information (per serving, 1 cup):- Calories:250- Protein: 6g- Carbohydrates: 15g- Fat: 20g- Fiber: 6g

67. CHICKPEA AND SPINACH STEW

Servings: 04 **Prep. time:** 10 minutes **Cook time:** 20 minutes

INGREDIENTS

- 1 tablespoon olive oil

- 1 medium onion, diced

- 3 garlic cloves, minced

- 1 teaspoon ground cumin

- 1/2 teaspoon smoked paprika

- 1/4 teaspoon red pepper flakes (optional)

- 1 can (15 oz) diced tomatoes

- 1 can (15 oz) chickpeas, drained and rinsed

- 4 cups fresh spinach

- Salt and pepper to taste

- 1/4 cup fresh cilantro, chopped

- Juice of 1/2 lemon

INSTRUCTIONS

1. Heat olive oil in a large skillet over medium heat. Add onion and sauté for 4-5 minutes until softened.

2. Add garlic, cumin, smoked paprika, and red pepper flakes (if using). Cook for 1-2 minutes until fragrant.

3. Stir in diced tomatoes and chickpeas. Simmer for 10 minutes, stirring occasionally.

4. Add spinach and cook for another 2-3 minutes until wilted. Season with salt, pepper, and lemon juice.

5. Garnish with fresh cilantro before serving.

Nutritional Information (per serving, 1 cup):- Calories:180- Protein: 6g- Carbohydrates: 22g- Fat: 6g- Fiber: 7g

Servings: 04   **Prep. time:** 10 minutes   **Cook time:** 00 minutes

INGREDIENTS

- 2 cups cooked chicken breast, shredded

- 1/2 cup Greek yogurt

- 1 tablespoon Dijon mustard

- 1 tablespoon lemon juice

- 1/4 cup celery, diced

- 1/4 cup red onion, diced

- 1/4 cup grapes, halved

- 1/4 cup walnuts, chopped

- Salt and pepper to taste

- Lettuce leaves or whole grain bread for serving

INSTRUCTIONS

1. In a large bowl, combine Greek yogurt, Dijon mustard, and lemon juice. Mix well.

2. Add shredded chicken, celery, red onion, grapes, walnuts, salt, and pepper. Stir until all ingredients are well coated.

3. Serve chilled on lettuce leaves or whole grain bread.

Nutritional Information (per serving, 1 cup):- Calories:200- Protein: 24g- Carbohydrates: 8g- Fat: 8g- Fiber:2g

Servings: 04   **Prep. time:** 10 minutes   **Cook time:** 10 minutes

INGREDIENTS

- 1 tablespoon sesame oil

- 1/2 cup onion, diced

- 2 garlic cloves, minced

- 1 cup bell peppers, diced (red, yellow, green)

- 2 cups cauliflower rice

- 1/2 cup frozen peas and carrots mix

- 2 tablespoons low-sodium soy sauce or tamari

- 1 tablespoon rice vinegar

- 1/4 teaspoon black pepper

- 2 large eggs, beaten

- 1/4 cup green onions, chopped

INSTRUCTIONS

1. 1. Heat sesame oil in a large skillet over medium-high heat. Add onion and garlic, and sauté for 3-4 minutes until softened.

2. Add bell peppers, cauliflower rice, peas, and carrots. Stir-fry for 5-7 minutes until vegetables are tender.

3. Stir in soy sauce, rice vinegar, and black pepper. Push vegetables to one side of the skillet and pour beaten eggs into the other side. Scramble the eggs until fully cooked.

4. Mix eggs with the vegetables. Garnish with green onions before serving.

Nutritional Information (per serving, 1 cup):- Calories:150- Protein: 7g- Carbohydrates: 12g- Fat: 9g- Fiber:4g

70. ROASTED BEET AND GOAT CHEESE SALAD

Servings: 04   **Prep. time:** 10 minutes   **Cook time:** 30 minutes

INGREDIENTS

- 4 medium beets, peeled and diced

- 2 tablespoons olive oil

- Salt and pepper to taste

- 4 cups mixed greens (arugula, spinach, etc.)

- 1/4 cup crumbled goat cheese

- 1/4 cup walnuts, toasted

- 1/4 cup balsamic vinaigrette

INSTRUCTIONS

1. Preheat the oven to 400°F (200°C). Toss diced beets with olive oil, salt, and pepper. Spread on a baking sheet and roast for 25-30 minutes, until tender.

2. In a large bowl, combine mixed greens, roasted beets, goat cheese, and walnuts.

3. Drizzle with balsamic vinaigrette and toss gently to combine. Serve immediately.

Nutritional Information (per serving, 1 cup):- Calories:220- Protein: 6g- Carbohydrates: 20g- Fat: 14g- Fiber:5g

Servings: 06   **Prep. time:** 10 minutes   **Cook time:** 35 minutes

INGREDIENTS

- 1 tablespoon olive oil

- 1 medium onion, diced

- 2 carrots, diced

- 2 celery stalks, diced

- 2 garlic cloves, minced

- 1 teaspoon ground cumin

- 1/2 teaspoon dried thyme

- 1 can (15 oz) diced tomatoes

- 1 cup dried green or brown lentils, rinsed

- 4 cups vegetable broth

- 2 cups kale, chopped

- Salt and pepper to taste

- 1 tablespoon lemon juice

INSTRUCTIONS

1. Heat olive oil in a large pot over medium heat. Add onion, carrots, and celery. Sauté for 5-6 minutes until softened.

2. Add garlic, cumin, and thyme, and cook for 1-2 minutes until fragrant.

3. Stir in diced tomatoes, lentils, and vegetable broth. Bring to a boil, then reduce heat and simmer for 25-30 minutes until lentils are tender.

4. Add kale and cook for another 5 minutes. Season with salt, pepper, and lemon juice.

5. Serve hot, garnished with extra lemon juice if desired.

Nutritional Information (per serving, 1 cup):- Calories:200- Protein: 10g- Carbohydrates: 30g- Fat: 5g- Fiber:12g

Servings: 04   **Prep. time:** 15 minutes   **Cook time:** 40 minutes

INGREDIENTS

- 4 bell peppers (red, yellow, green, or orange)

- 1 cup quinoa, rinsed

- 2 cups vegetable broth

- 1 tablespoon olive oil

- 1 small onion, diced

- 2 garlic cloves, minced

- 1 zucchini, diced

- 1 cup cherry tomatoes, halved

- 1 cup black beans, drained and rinsed

- 1 teaspoon ground cumin

- 1/2 teaspoon smoked paprika

- Salt and pepper to taste

- 1/2 cup shredded mozzarella cheese (optional)

- Fresh cilantro, chopped (for garnish)

INSTRUCTIONS

1. Preheat the oven to 375°F (190°C). Cut the tops off the bell peppers and remove seeds. Place them in a baking dish, cut side up.

2. In a medium saucepan, bring vegetable broth to a boil. Add quinoa, reduce heat, cover, and simmer for 15 minutes or until quinoa is cooked and fluffy.

3. In a skillet, heat olive oil over medium heat. Sauté onion and garlic for 3-4 minutes until softened. Add zucchini, cherry tomatoes, black beans, cumin, smoked paprika, salt, and pepper. Cook for 5-7 minutes until vegetables are tender.

4. Stir in the cooked quinoa and mix well.

5. Stuff each bell pepper with the quinoa-vegetable mixture. Top with mozzarella cheese if desired.

6. Cover the dish with foil and bake for 30 minutes. Remove foil and bake for an additional 10 minutes until the peppers are tender and cheese is melted.

7. Garnish with fresh cilantro and serve hot.

Nutritional Information (per pepper):- Calories:280- Protein: 10g- Carbohydrates: 45g- Fat: 8g- Fiber:9g

Servings: 04   **Prep. time:** 15 minutes   **Cook time:** 30 minutes

INGREDIENTS

- 4 boneless, skinless chicken breasts

- Salt and pepper to taste

- 1 tablespoon olive oil

- 1 cup fresh spinach, chopped

- 1/4 cup sun-dried tomatoes, chopped

- 1/2 cup crumbled feta cheese

- 1 teaspoon dried oregano

- 1/2 teaspoon garlic powder

- Toothpicks

INSTRUCTIONS

1. Preheat the oven to 375°F (190°C). Slice a pocket into each chicken breast by cutting horizontally without going all the way through. Season with salt and pepper.

2. In a skillet, heat olive oil over medium heat. Add spinach and sauté for 2-3 minutes until wilted. Remove from heat and mix in sun-dried tomatoes, feta cheese, oregano, and garlic powder.

3. Stuff each chicken breast with the spinach mixture and secure with toothpicks.

4. Place stuffed chicken breasts on a baking sheet lined with parchment paper.

5. Bake for 25-30 minutes, or until the chicken is cooked through and the internal temperature reaches 165°F (74°C).

6. Remove toothpicks and serve hot with a side of vegetables or a salad.

Nutritional Information (per chicken breast):- Calories:300- Protein: 36g- Carbohydrates: 4g- Fat: 16g- Fiber:1g

Servings: 04   **Prep. time:** 10 minutes   **Cook time:** 30 minutes

INGREDIENTS

- 1 tablespoon coconut oil

- 1 large onion, diced

- 3 garlic cloves, minced

- 1 tablespoon fresh ginger, grated

- 2 teaspoons curry powder

- 1/2 teaspoon turmeric powder

- 1/2 teaspoon ground cumin

- 1/4 teaspoon cayenne pepper (optional)

- 1 can (14 oz) coconut milk

- 1 1/2 cups vegetable broth

- 2 large sweet potatoes, peeled and diced

- 1 cup dried red lentils, rinsed

- Salt and pepper to taste

- 2 cups fresh spinach

- 1/4 cup fresh cilantro, chopped (for garnish)

INSTRUCTIONS

1. In a large pot, heat coconut oil over medium heat. Add onion and sauté for 5-6 minutes until softened.

2. Add garlic, ginger, curry powder, turmeric, cumin, and cayenne pepper (if using). Cook for 1-2 minutes until fragrant.

3. Pour in coconut milk and vegetable broth. Add sweet potatoes and lentils. Bring to a boil, then reduce heat and simmer for 20-25 minutes until sweet potatoes are tender and lentils are cooked through.

4. Stir in fresh spinach and cook for another 2-3 minutes until wilted. Season with salt and pepper.

5. Serve hot, garnished with fresh cilantro and with a side of rice or naan bread.

Nutritional Information (per serving, 1 cup):- Calories:320- Protein: 10g- Carbohydrates: 50g- Fat: 12g- Fiber:12g

Servings: 04   **Prep. time:** 05 minutes   **Chill time:** 4 hours

INGREDIENTS

- 1/2 cup chia seeds

- 2 cups unsweetened coconut milk

- 1 tablespoon maple syrup or honey

- 1 teaspoon vanilla extract

- 1 ripe mango, diced

- 1/4 cup shredded unsweetened coconut

- Fresh mint leaves (for garnish)

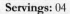

INSTRUCTIONS

1. In a medium bowl, combine chia seeds, coconut milk, maple syrup, and vanilla extract. Stir well to combine.

2. Cover and refrigerate for at least 4 hours or overnight, until the chia seeds have absorbed the liquid and the mixture is thickened.

3. When ready to serve, divide the chia pudding into bowls or jars. Top with diced mango and shredded coconut.

4. Garnish with fresh mint leaves and serve cold.

Nutritional Information (per serving, 1/2 cup):- Calories:210- Protein: 4g- Carbohydrates: 20g- Fat: 14g- Fiber:8g

Servings: 04   **Prep. time:** 10 minutes   **Cook time:** 00 minutes

INGREDIENTS

- 4 salmon fillets

- 1 tablespoon olive oil

- Salt and pepper to taste

- 1/2 cup Greek yogurt

- 1 tablespoon fresh dill, chopped

- 1 tablespoon lemon juice

- 1 teaspoon lemon zest

- 1 garlic clove, minced

INSTRUCTIONS

1. Preheat the grill to medium-high heat. Brush salmon fillets with olive oil and season with salt and pepper.

2. Grill salmon for 4-5 minutes per side, until cooked through and flaky.

3. In a small bowl, mix Greek yogurt, dill, lemon juice, lemon zest, and minced garlic. Stir well to combine.

4. Serve grilled salmon with a dollop of lemon-dill yogurt sauce on top. Pair with a side of steamed vegetables or a quinoa salad.

Nutritional Information (per fillet with sauce):- Calories:300- Protein: 34g- Carbohydrates: 2g- Fat: 18g- Fiber:0g

Servings: 02   **Prep. time:** 05 minutes   **Cook time:** 4 hours

INGREDIENTS

- 1 cup rolled oats

- 1 cup unsweetened almond milk

- 1/2 cup unsweetened applesauce

- 1 tablespoon chia seeds

- 1 teaspoon ground cinnamon

- 1 tablespoon maple syrup or honey

- 1/4 cup chopped walnuts

- 1/2 apple, diced

INSTRUCTIONS

1. In a mason jar or airtight container, combine oats, almond milk, applesauce, chia seeds, cinnamon, and maple syrup. Stir well.
2. Cover and refrigerate overnight or for at least 4 hours.
3. When ready to serve, top with chopped walnuts and diced apple.

Nutritional Information (per serving, 1 cup):- Calories:280- Protein: 7g- Carbohydrates: 44g- Fat: 10g- Fiber:8g

78. CAULIFLOWER CRUST PIZZA WITH VEGGIES

Servings: 04   **Prep. time:** 15 minutes   **Cook time:** 25 minutes

INGREDIENTS

- 1 medium head of cauliflower, chopped

- 1/2 cup shredded mozzarella cheese

- 1/4 cup grated Parmesan cheese

- 1/2 teaspoon dried oregano

- 1/4 teaspoon garlic powder

- 1/4 teaspoon salt

- 1 large egg

- 1/2 cup tomato sauce

- 1/2 cup bell peppers, sliced

- 1/2 cup mushrooms, sliced

- 1/4 cup red onion, thinly sliced

- 1/2 cup cherry tomatoes, halved

- Fresh basil leaves (for garnish)

INSTRUCTIONS

1. Preheat the oven to 425°F (220°C). Line a baking sheet with parchment paper.

2. In a food processor, pulse cauliflower until it resembles rice. Transfer to a microwave-safe bowl and microwave for 5 minutes. Let cool slightly, then place in a clean kitchen towel and squeeze out excess moisture.

3. In a bowl, mix cauliflower, mozzarella, Parmesan, oregano, garlic powder, salt, and egg until well combined.

4. Spread the mixture into a circle on the prepared baking sheet, about 1/4-inch thick. Bake for 10-12 minutes until golden and firm.

5. Spread tomato sauce over the crust, then top with bell peppers, mushrooms, red onion, and cherry tomatoes.

6. Bake for another 10-12 minutes until the vegetables are tender.

7. Garnish with fresh basil leaves and serve hot.

Nutritional Information (per slice, 1/4 of pizza):- Calories:150- Protein: 8g- Carbohydrates: 12g- Fat: 8g- Fiber:3g

Servings: 12   **Prep. time:** 10 minutes   **Cook time:** 20 minutes

INGREDIENTS

- 1 medium head of cauliflower, chopped

- 1/2 cup shredded mozzarella cheese

- 1/4 cup grated Parmesan cheese

- 1/2 teaspoon dried oregano

- 1/4 teaspoon garlic powder

- 1/4 teaspoon salt

- 1 large egg

- 1/2 cup tomato sauce

- 1/2 cup bell peppers, sliced

- 1/2 cup mushrooms, sliced

- 1/4 cup red onion, thinly sliced

- 1/2 cup cherry tomatoes, halved

- Fresh basil leaves (for garnish)

INSTRUCTIONS

1. Preheat the oven to 350°F (175°C). Grease a 12-cup muffin tin with olive oil.

2. In a large bowl, whisk together eggs, milk, salt, and pepper.

3. Add broccoli, cheddar cheese, bell pepper, and green onions. Mix well.

4. Pour the egg mixture evenly into the muffin tin cups.

5. Bake for 18-20 minutes until the egg muffins are set and slightly golden.

6. Let cool for a few minutes before removing from the muffin tin. Serve warm or cold.

Nutritional Information (per muffin):- Calories:80- Protein: 6g- Carbohydrates: 2g- Fat: 6g- Fiber:1g

Servings: 04   **Prep. time:** 10 minutes   **Cook time:** 00 minutes

INGREDIENTS

- 1 can (15 oz) chickpeas, drained and rinsed

- 1 cup cucumber, diced

- 1 cup cherry tomatoes, halved

- 1/4 cup red onion, finely chopped

- 1/4 cup Kalamata olives, sliced

- 1/4 cup feta cheese, crumbled

- 2 tablespoons olive oil

- 1 tablespoon red wine vinegar

- 1 tablespoon lemon juice

- 1 teaspoon dried oregano

- Salt and pepper to taste

INSTRUCTIONS

1. In a large bowl, combine chickpeas, cucumber, cherry tomatoes, red onion, olives, and feta cheese.

2. In a small bowl, whisk together olive oil, red wine vinegar, lemon juice, oregano, salt, and pepper.

3. Pour the dressing over the salad and toss to coat. Serve immediately or chill for an hour for enhanced flavors.

Nutritional Information (per serving, 1 cup):- Calories:200- Protein: 6g- Carbohydrates: 20g- Fat: 12g-Fiber:6g

Servings: 8 tacos   **Prep. time:** 10 minutes   **Cook time:** 25 minutes

INGREDIENTS

- 2 medium sweet potatoes, peeled and diced

- 1 tablespoon olive oil

- 1/2 teaspoon chili powder

- 1/2 teaspoon cumin

- Salt and pepper to taste

- 1 can (15 oz) black beans, drained and rinsed

- 8 small corn tortillas

- 1/2 cup shredded lettuce

- 1/4 cup red onion, diced

- 1/4 cup cilantro, chopped

- 1/4 cup crumbled cotija or feta cheese

- Lime wedges (for serving)

INSTRUCTIONS

1. Preheat oven to 400°F (200°C). Toss diced sweet potatoes with olive oil, chili powder, cumin, salt, and pepper. Spread on a baking sheet and roast for 20-25 minutes until tender.

2. In a small pot, warm black beans over low heat until heated through.

3. Warm tortillas in a skillet over medium heat or directly over a gas flame for a few seconds until soft.

4. Assemble tacos by adding roasted sweet potatoes, black beans, lettuce, red onion, cilantro, and cheese to each tortilla.

5. Serve with lime wedges.

Nutritional Information (per taco):- Calories:150- Protein: 5g- Carbohydrates: 28g- Fat: 4g- Fiber:7g

Servings: 04   **Prep. time:** 10 minutes   **Cook time:** 30 minutes

INGREDIENTS

- 1 tablespoon olive oil

- 1 large onion, chopped

- 2 garlic cloves, minced

- 1 tablespoon fresh ginger, grated

- 6 large carrots, peeled and sliced

- 4 cups vegetable broth

- 1/2 cup coconut milk

- Salt and pepper to taste

- Fresh cilantro, chopped (for garnish)

INSTRUCTIONS

1. In a large pot, heat olive oil over medium heat. Add onion and sauté for 5-6 minutes until softened.

2. Add garlic and ginger and cook for another 1-2 minutes until fragrant.

3. Add carrots and vegetable broth. Bring to a boil, then reduce heat and simmer for 20-25 minutes until carrots are tender.

4. Use an immersion blender to puree the soup until smooth. Stir in coconut milk and season with salt and pepper.

5. Serve hot, garnished with fresh cilantro.

Nutritional Information (per serving, 1 cup):- Calories:120- Protein: 2g- Carbohydrates: 16g- Fat: 6g- Fiber:3g

Servings: 04   **Prep. time:** 15 minutes   **Cook time:** 45 minutes

INGREDIENTS

- 1 large eggplant, sliced into 1/2-inch rounds

- 1 tablespoon salt

- 1 cup whole wheat breadcrumbs

- 1/4 cup grated Parmesan cheese

- 1 teaspoon Italian seasoning

- 2 large eggs, beaten

- 2 cups marinara sauce

- 1 1/2 cups shredded mozzarella cheese

- Fresh basil leaves (for garnish)

INSTRUCTIONS

1. Preheat the oven to 375°F (190°C). Arrange eggplant slices on a baking sheet and sprinkle with salt. Let sit for 15 minutes to draw out moisture, then rinse and pat dry.

2. In a bowl, combine breadcrumbs, Parmesan cheese, and Italian seasoning. Dip each eggplant slice in beaten eggs, then coat with the breadcrumb mixture.

3. Arrange eggplant slices on a baking sheet and bake for 20 minutes, flipping halfway through, until golden.

4. In a baking dish, layer baked eggplant slices, marinara sauce, and mozzarella cheese. Repeat until all ingredients are used, ending with cheese on top.

5. Bake for 20-25 minutes until cheese is melted and bubbly.

6. Garnish with fresh basil leaves and serve hot.

Nutritional Information (per serving, 1 cup):- Calories:300- Protein: 15g- Carbohydrates: 28g- Fat: 16g- Fiber:6g

Servings: 8 wraps   **Prep. time:** 10 minutes   **Cook time:** 15 minutes

INGREDIENTS

- 1 lb ground chicken

- 1 tablespoon olive oil

- 2 garlic cloves, minced

- 1 small onion, diced

- 1 red bell pepper, diced

- 1/4 cup grated carrots

- 1/4 cup hoisin sauce

- 2 tablespoons peanut butter

- 1 tablespoon soy sauce

- 1 tablespoon rice vinegar

- 1 teaspoon sriracha (optional)

- 8 large lettuce leaves (like Bibb or Romaine)

- 1/4 cup chopped peanuts

- 2 tablespoons fresh cilantro, chopped

INSTRUCTIONS

1. In a large skillet, heat olive oil over medium heat. Add garlic and onion, and sauté for 3-4 minutes until softened.

2. Add ground chicken and cook, breaking it apart with a spoon, until browned and cooked through, about 6-8 minutes.

3. Stir in bell pepper and carrots, and cook for another 3-4 minutes.

4. In a small bowl, mix hoisin sauce, peanut butter, soy sauce, rice vinegar, and sriracha. Pour over the chicken mixture and stir to coat. Cook for another 2-3 minutes.

5. Serve chicken mixture in lettuce leaves, topped with chopped peanuts and cilantro.

Nutritional Information (per wrap):- Calories:150- Protein: 14g- Carbohydrates: 7g- Fat: 8g- Fiber:1g

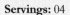

Servings: 04   **Prep. time:** 10 minutes   **Cook time:** 10 minutes

INGREDIENTS

- 4 medium zucchinis, spiralized into noodles

- 2 tablespoons olive oil

- 2 cups cherry tomatoes, halved

- 1/2 cup homemade or store-bought pesto

- Salt and pepper to taste

- 1/4 cup pine nuts, toasted

- 1/4 cup Parmesan cheese, grated (optional)

INSTRUCTIONS

1. Heat olive oil in a large skillet over medium heat. Add cherry tomatoes and cook for 4-5 minutes until softened.

2. Add zucchini noodles to the skillet and sauté for 2-3 minutes until just tender but still firm.

3. Remove from heat and toss with pesto. Season with salt and pepper.

4. Serve topped with toasted pine nuts and Parmesan cheese, if desired.

Nutritional Information (per wrap):- Calories:150- Protein: 14g- Carbohydrates: 7g- Fat: 8g- Fiber:1g

Servings: 04   **Prep. time:** 10 minutes   **Cook time:** 00 minutes

INGREDIENTS

- 1 can (15 oz) chickpeas, drained and rinsed

- 1 ripe avocado

- 1/4 cup red onion, finely chopped

- 1/4 cup celery, finely chopped

- 1 tablespoon lemon juice

- Salt and pepper to taste

- 4 slices whole grain bread

- 1/2 cup baby spinach leaves

INSTRUCTIONS

1. In a bowl, mash chickpeas and avocado together until combined but still slightly chunky.

2. Stir in red onion, celery, lemon juice, salt, and pepper.

3. Spread the mixture on two slices of whole grain bread. Top with spinach leaves and the remaining slices of bread.

4. Serve immediately or pack for lunch.

Nutritional Information (per sandwich):- Calories:320- Protein: 10g- Carbohydrates: 42g- Fat: 14g- Fiber:10g

Servings: 04   **Prep. time:** 10 minutes   **Cook time:** 00 minutes

INGREDIENTS

- 2 cups cooked chicken breast, shredded

- 1/2 cup plain Greek yogurt

- 1 tablespoon Dijon mustard

- 1 tablespoon lemon juice

- 1/4 cup celery, diced

- 1/4 cup red grapes, halved

- 2 tablespoons slivered almonds

- Salt and pepper to taste

- 4 leaves Romaine lettuce (for serving)

INSTRUCTIONS

1. In a large bowl, combine shredded chicken, Greek yogurt, Dijon mustard, lemon juice, celery, grapes, and almonds. Mix until well combined.

2. Season with salt and pepper to taste.

3. Serve the chicken salad in lettuce leaves or on whole grain bread.

Nutritional Information (per serving, 1/2 cup):- Calories:160- Protein: 25g- Carbohydrates: 5g- Fat:4g- Fiber:1g

Servings: 04   **Prep. time:** 10 minutes   **Cook time:** 15 minutes

INGREDIENTS

- 1 medium head of cauliflower, chopped into florets

- 1 tablespoon sesame oil

- 2 garlic cloves, minced

- 1 small onion, diced

- 1 cup frozen peas and carrots

- 2 large eggs, beaten

- 3 tablespoons low-sodium soy sauce

- 1 tablespoon hoisin sauce (optional)

- 2 green onions, sliced

- 1 tablespoon sesame seeds (for garnish)

INSTRUCTIONS

1. Pulse cauliflower in a food processor until it resembles rice.
2. Heat sesame oil in a large skillet over medium heat. Add garlic and onion and sauté for 3-4 minutes.
3. Add peas and carrots and cook for another 3 minutes.
4. Push vegetables to one side of the skillet. Pour in beaten eggs on the other side and scramble until fully cooked.
5. Stir in cauliflower rice, soy sauce, and hoisin sauce (if using). Cook for 5-7 minutes until cauliflower is tender.
6. Garnish with green onions and sesame seeds before serving.

Nutritional Information (per serving, 1 cup):- Calories:120- Protein: 5g- Carbohydrates: 15g- Fat:5g- Fiber:4g

89. LENTIL AND SPINACH STEW

Servings: 04   **Prep. time:** 10 minutes   **Cook time:** 30 minutes

INGREDIENTS

- 1 tablespoon olive oil

- 1 large onion, diced

- 2 garlic cloves, minced

- 1 cup dried green or brown lentils, rinsed

- 4 cups vegetable broth

- 1 can (14 oz) diced tomatoes

- 1 teaspoon ground cumin

- 1/2 teaspoon smoked paprika

- Salt and pepper to taste

- 4 cups fresh spinach

- 1/4 cup fresh parsley, chopped (for garnish)

INSTRUCTIONS

1. In a large pot, heat olive oil over medium heat. Add onion and sauté for 5-6 minutes until softened.

2. Add garlic and cook for another 1-2 minutes until fragrant.

3. Add lentils, vegetable broth, diced tomatoes, cumin, smoked paprika, salt, and pepper. Bring to a boil, then reduce heat and simmer for 25-30 minutes until lentils are tender.

4. Stir in spinach and cook for another 2-3 minutes until wilted.

5. Serve hot, garnished with fresh parsley.

Nutritional Information (per serving, 1 cup):- Calories:180- Protein: 12g- Carbohydrates: 30g- Fat:3g- Fiber:12g

Servings: 12 tablespoons   **Prep. time:** 05 minutes   **Cook time:** 10 minutes

INGREDIENTS

- 2 cups fresh or frozen blueberries

- 2 tablespoons chia seeds

- 1-2 tablespoons maple syrup (optional)

- 1/2 teaspoon vanilla extract

INSTRUCTIONS

1. In a medium saucepan, cook blueberries over medium heat for about 5 minutes until they begin to break down, stirring occasionally.

2. Mash blueberries with a fork or potato masher to your desired consistency.

3. Stir in chia seeds, maple syrup (if using), and vanilla extract. Cook for another 5 minutes until the jam thickens.

4. Remove from heat and let cool. Store in an airtight container in the refrigerator for up to 1 week.

Nutritional Information (per tablespoon):- Calories:15- Protein: 0.3g- Carbohydrates: 3g- Fat:0.3g- Fiber:1g

91. SPICY QUINOA AND BLACK BEAN STUFFED PEPPERS

Servings: 8 stuffed pepper halves

Prep. time: 15 minutes

Cook time: 30 minutes

INGREDIENTS

- 4 large bell peppers, halved and seeds removed

- 1 cup quinoa, rinsed

- 2 cups vegetable broth

- 1 tablespoon olive oil

- 1 small onion, diced

- 2 garlic cloves, minced

- 1 can (15 oz) black beans, drained and rinsed

- 1 cup corn kernels (fresh or frozen)

- 1 teaspoon chili powder

- 1/2 teaspoon cumin

- Salt and pepper to taste

- 1/2 cup shredded cheddar cheese

- 1/4 cup chopped cilantro (for garnish)

INSTRUCTIONS

1. Preheat the oven to 375°F (190°C). Place bell pepper halves in a baking dish, cut side up.

2. In a medium saucepan, bring quinoa and vegetable broth to a boil. Reduce heat to low, cover, and simmer for 15 minutes until quinoa is cooked.

3. In a skillet, heat olive oil over medium heat. Sauté onion and garlic for 3-4 minutes until softened.

4. Add black beans, corn, chili powder, cumin, salt, and pepper. Cook for 5 minutes, then stir in cooked quinoa.

5. Fill each bell pepper half with the quinoa mixture and top with shredded cheese.

6. Cover the baking dish with aluminum foil and bake for 25 minutes. Remove foil and bake for an additional 5 minutes until cheese is melted and bubbly.

7. Garnish with chopped cilantro and serve.

Nutritional Information (per pepper half):- Calories:200- Protein: 8g- Carbohydrates: 34g- Fat:5g- Fiber:7g

92. ALMOND BUTTER BANANA SMOOTHIE

Servings: 01   **Prep. time:** 05 minutes   **Cook time:** 00 minutes

INGREDIENTS

- 1 ripe banana

- 1 cup unsweetened almond milk

- 2 tablespoons almond butter

- 1 tablespoon chia seeds

- 1/2 teaspoon vanilla extract

- 1/2 cup ice cubes

INSTRUCTIONS

1. Combine all ingredients in a blender and blend until smooth.

2. Pour into a glass and serve immediately.

Nutritional Information (per serving):- Calories: 250- Protein: 5g- Carbohydrates: 34g- Fat: 11g- Fiber: 6g

93. SWEET POTATO AND KALE HASH

Servings: 04   **Prep. time:** 10 minutes   **Cook time:** 20 minutes

INGREDIENTS

- 1 ripe banana

- 1 cup unsweetened almond milk

- 2 tablespoons almond butter

- 1 tablespoon chia seeds

- 1/2 teaspoon vanilla extract

- 1/2 cup ice cubes

INSTRUCTIONS

1. Heat olive oil in a large skillet over medium heat. Add sweet potato and cook for 8-10 minutes, stirring occasionally until tender.

2. Add onion and bell pepper, and sauté for another 5 minutes until softened.

3. Stir in kale, garlic, salt, pepper, and smoked paprika. Cook for another 3-4 minutes until kale is wilted.

4. Make four small wells in the hash and crack an egg into each well. Cover and cook for 4-5 minutes until eggs are cooked to your liking.

5. Serve hot, with a sprinkle of salt and pepper on the eggs.

Nutritional Information (per serving, 1/4 of hash with an egg):- Calories: 230- Protein: 8g- Carbohydrates: 20g- Fat: 12g- Fiber: 5g

Servings: 04   **Prep. time:** 10 minutes   **Cook time:** 25 minutes

INGREDIENTS

- 4 boneless, skinless chicken breasts

- 1 tablespoon olive oil

- Salt and pepper to taste

- 1 teaspoon dried oregano

- 1/2 cup fresh spinach, chopped

- 1/4 cup feta cheese, crumbled

- 2 garlic cloves, minced

- 1/4 cup sun-dried tomatoes, chopped

INSTRUCTIONS

1. Preheat the oven to 375°F (190°C). Cut a pocket in each chicken breast, being careful not to cut all the way through.

2. In a bowl, mix spinach, feta cheese, garlic, and sun-dried tomatoes.

3. Stuff each chicken breast with the spinach mixture and secure with toothpicks.

4. Season the chicken with salt, pepper, and oregano. Heat olive oil in a large oven-safe skillet over medium-high heat.

5. Sear chicken for 3-4 minutes per side until golden. Transfer the skillet to the oven and bake for 15-20 minutes until the chicken is cooked through.

6. Remove toothpicks before serving.

Nutritional Information (per serving, 1 chicken breast):- Calories: 300- Protein: 35g- Carbohydrates: 3g- Fat: 17g- Fiber: 1g

Servings: 04   **Prep. time:** 10 minutes   **Cook time:** 05 minutes

INGREDIENTS

- 1 cup whole wheat couscous

- 1 1/4 cups vegetable broth

- 1/2 cup cucumber, diced

- 1/2 cup cherry tomatoes, halved

- 1/4 cup Kalamata olives, sliced

- 1/4 cup red onion, finely chopped

- 1/4 cup feta cheese, crumbled

- 2 tablespoons fresh parsley, chopped

- 2 tablespoons olive oil

- 1 tablespoon lemon juice

- Salt and pepper to taste

INSTRUCTIONS

1. Bring vegetable broth to a boil in a medium saucepan. Remove from heat, stir in couscous, cover, and let stand for 5 minutes. Fluff with a fork and let cool.

2. In a large bowl, combine cooled couscous, cucumber, cherry tomatoes, olives, red onion, feta cheese, and parsley.

3. In a small bowl, whisk together olive oil, lemon juice, salt, and pepper. Pour over salad and toss to coat.

4. Serve chilled or at room temperature.

Nutritional Information (per serving, 1 cup):- Calories: 220- Protein: 6g- Carbohydrates: 30g- Fat: 9g- Fiber: 4g

Servings: 04   **Prep. time:** 10 minutes   **Cook time:** 25 minutes

INGREDIENTS

- 1 lb Brussels sprouts, trimmed and halved

- 2 tablespoons olive oil

- Salt and pepper to taste

- 1/4 cup balsamic vinegar

- 1 tablespoon honey

INSTRUCTIONS

1. Preheat the oven to 400°F (200°C). Toss Brussels sprouts with olive oil, salt, and pepper.

2. Spread on a baking sheet and roast for 20-25 minutes, stirring halfway through, until tender and caramelized.

3. Meanwhile, in a small saucepan, simmer balsamic vinegar and honey over medium heat for 5-7 minutes until reduced and thickened.

4. Drizzle balsamic glaze over roasted Brussels sprouts before serving.

Nutritional Information (per serving, 1/2 cup):- Calories: 100- Protein: 2g- Carbohydrates: 14g- Fat: 5g- Fiber: 4g

97. CHIA SEED PUDDING WITH FRESH BERRIES

Servings: 02   **Prep. time:** 05 minutes   **Chill time:** 4 hours

INGREDIENTS

- 1/4 cup chia seeds

- 1 cup unsweetened almond milk

- 1 tablespoon maple syrup

- 1/2 teaspoon vanilla extract

-1/2 cup mixed fresh berries
(blueberries,strawberries,
raspberries)

INSTRUCTIONS

1. In a bowl, whisk together chia seeds, almond milk, maple syrup, and vanilla extract.

2. Cover and refrigerate for at least 4 hours or overnight until thickened.

3. Serve topped with fresh berries.

Nutritional Information (per serving, 1/2 cup):- Calories: 150- Protein: 4g- Carbohydrates: 20g- Fat: 7g- Fiber: 8g

Servings: 02   **Prep. time:** 10 minutes   **Cook time:** 06 minutes

INGREDIENTS

- 1 lb large shrimp, peeled and deveined

- 1 tablespoon olive oil

- Salt and pepper to taste

- 4 cups mixed salad greens

- 1 ripe avocado, diced

- 1/2 cup cherry tomatoes, halved

- 1/4 cup red onion, thinly sliced

- 1/4 cup cilantro, chopped

LIME DRESSING

- 2 tablespoons lime juice

- 1 tablespoon olive oil

- 1 teaspoon honey

- Salt and pepper to taste

INSTRUCTIONS

1. Heat olive oil in a large skillet over medium heat. Season shrimp with salt and pepper. Cook for 2-3 minutes on each side until opaque and pink. Remove from heat and let cool.

2. In a large bowl, combine salad greens, avocado, cherry tomatoes, red onion, and cilantro.

3. Whisk together lime juice, olive oil, honey, salt, and pepper in a small bowl.

4. Add shrimp to the salad and drizzle with lime dressing. Toss gently to combine. Serve immediately.

Nutritional Information (per serving, 1/2 salad):- Calories: 300- Protein: 28g- Carbohydrates: 12g- Fat: 17g- Fiber: 5g

Servings: 02   **Prep. time:** 10 minutes   **Cook time:** 06 minutes

INGREDIENTS

- 1 medium head cauliflower, cut into florets

- 1/2 cup shredded mozzarella cheese

- 1/4 cup grated Parmesan cheese

- 1 large egg, beaten

- 1/2 teaspoon dried oregano

- Salt and pepper to taste

- 1/2 cup marinara sauce

- 1/2 cup fresh mozzarella cheese, sliced

- 1/4 cup fresh basil leaves

INSTRUCTIONS

1. Preheat the oven to 425°F (220°C). Line a baking sheet with parchment paper.

2. Pulse cauliflower in a food processor until it resembles rice. Transfer to a microwave-safe bowl and microwave for 5-6 minutes until soft. Let cool slightly, then squeeze out excess moisture using a clean kitchen towel.

3. In a bowl, combine cauliflower, shredded mozzarella, Parmesan, egg, oregano, salt, and pepper. Mix well to form a dough.

4. Spread cauliflower dough onto the prepared baking sheet in a 10-inch circle. Bake for 12-15 minutes until golden and crisp.

5. Spread marinara sauce over the crust, top with fresh mozzarella slices, and bake for an additional 7-10 minutes until cheese is melted and bubbly.

6. Garnish with fresh basil leaves before serving.

Nutritional Information (per slice, 1/4 of pizza):- Calories: 180- Protein: 12g- Carbohydrates: 10g- Fat: 10g- Fiber: 2g

Servings: 06   **Prep. time:** 10 minutes   **Cook time:** 30 minutes

INGREDIENTS

- 1 tablespoon olive oil

- 1 large onion, diced

- 3 garlic cloves, minced

- 1 teaspoon ground cumin

- 1 teaspoon ground coriander

- 1/2 teaspoon smoked paprika

- 1/4 teaspoon cayenne pepper

- 1 can (15 oz) chickpeas, drained and rinsed

- 1 cup dried red lentils, rinsed

- 1 can (14 oz) diced tomatoes

- 4 cups vegetable broth

- Salt and pepper to taste

- 2 cups spinach, chopped

- 1/4 cup fresh cilantro, chopped (for garnish)

INSTRUCTIONS

1. Heat olive oil in a large pot over medium heat. Add onion and cook for 5-6 minutes until softened. Add garlic and spices, and cook for another 1-2 minutes.

2. Stir in chickpeas, lentils, diced tomatoes, vegetable broth, salt, and pepper. Bring to a boil, then reduce heat and simmer for 25-30 minutes until lentils are tender.

3. Stir in spinach and cook for another 2-3 minutes until wilted.

4. Serve hot, garnished with fresh cilantro.

Nutritional Information (per serving, 1 cup):- Calories: 220- Protein: 12g- Carbohydrates: 34g- Fat: 4g- Fiber: 10g

Servings: 04   **Prep. time:** 10 minutes   **Cook time:** 00 minutes

INGREDIENTS

- 2 cups plain Greek yogurt

- 1/2 cup granola (preferably low-sugar)

- 1 cup mixed berries (blueberries, strawberries, raspberries)

- 2 tablespoons honey

- 1 tablespoon chia seeds (optional)

INSTRUCTIONS

1. In four serving glasses, layer 1/2 cup Greek yogurt, 2 tablespoons granola, and 1/4 cup berries.

2. Drizzle with honey and sprinkle with chia seeds if using.

3. Repeat layers, ending with berries on top. Serve immediately.

Nutritional Information (per serving, 1 parfait):- Calories: 250- Protein: 14g- Carbohydrates: 36g- Fat: 6g- Fiber: 4g

Servings: 06   **Prep. time:** 10 minutes   **Cook time:** 30 minutes

INGREDIENTS

- 1 tablespoon coconut oil

- 1 large onion, diced

- 2 garlic cloves, minced

- 1 tablespoon fresh ginger, minced

- 1 tablespoon curry powder

- 1/2 teaspoon turmeric

- 1/4 teaspoon cinnamon

- 1 large sweet potato, peeled and diced

- 1 cup dried green or brown lentils, rinsed

- 4 cups vegetable broth

- 1 can (14 oz) coconut milk

- 2 cups kale, chopped

- Salt and pepper to taste

INSTRUCTIONS

1. Heat coconut oil in a large pot over medium heat. Add onion and sauté for 5-6 minutes until softened.

2. Add garlic, ginger, curry powder, turmeric, and cinnamon. Cook for 1-2 minutes until fragrant.

3. Add sweet potato, lentils, vegetable broth, and coconut milk. Bring to a boil, then reduce heat and simmer for 25-30 minutes until lentils and sweet potatoes are tender.

4. Stir in kale and cook for another 2-3 minutes until wilted. Season with salt and pepper to taste. Serve hot.

Nutritional Information (per serving, 1 cup):- Calories: 260- Protein: 10g- Carbohydrates: 36g- Fat: 10g- Fiber: 8g

Servings: 04   **Prep. time:** 10 minutes   **Cook time:** 30 minutes

INGREDIENTS

- 1 large eggplant, diced

- 2 tablespoons olive oil

- 1 small onion, diced

- 2 celery stalks, diced

- 2 garlic cloves, minced

- 1/2 cup green olives, sliced

- 1/4 cup capers, rinsed

- 1 can (14 oz) diced tomatoes

- 1 tablespoon red wine vinegar

- 1 tablespoon honey

- Salt and pepper to taste

- 1/4 cup fresh basil, chopped

INSTRUCTIONS

1. Heat olive oil in a large skillet over medium heat. Add eggplant and cook for 8-10 minutes until softened.

2. Add onion, celery, and garlic, and cook for another 5 minutes.

3. Stir in olives, capers, diced tomatoes, vinegar, honey, salt, and pepper. Simmer for 15-20 minutes until flavors meld and the mixture thickens.

4. Remove from heat and stir in fresh basil. Serve warm or at room temperature.

Nutritional Information (per serving, 1/2 cup):- Calories: 120- Protein: 2g- Carbohydrates: 17g- Fat: 6g- Fiber: 5g

104. APPLE CINNAMON OVERNIGHT OATS

Servings: 02   **Prep. time:** 05 minutes   **Chill time:** 4 hours

INGREDIENTS

- 1 cup rolled oats

- 1 cup unsweetened almond milk

- 1/2 cup unsweetened applesauce

- 1/2 teaspoon ground cinnamon

- 1 tablespoon chia seeds

- 1 tablespoon maple syrup

- 1/2 cup chopped apples

- 1/4 cup walnuts, chopped (optional)

INSTRUCTIONS

1. In a mason jar or airtight container, mix oats, almond milk, applesauce, cinnamon, chia seeds, and maple syrup. Stir well to combine.

2. Cover and refrigerate overnight or for at least 4 hours.

3. Top with chopped apples and walnuts before serving.

Nutritional Information (per serving, 1 parfait):- Calories: 220- Protein: 6g- Carbohydrates: 36g- Fat: 7g- Fiber: 6g

30-DAY MEAL PLAN STRATEGIES

Below is a 30-day meal plan table using the recipes from "The Good Energy Cookbook." The plan is balanced, providing a variety of breakfast, lunch, dinner, and snack options, incorporating all recipe categories (breakfast, first courses, meat and fish main courses, side dishes, and desserts). This meal plan is designed to support metabolic health, weight management, and overall wellness, inspired by Dr. Casey Means' approach.

Day	Breakfast	Lunch	Dinner	Snack/Dessert
1	Chia Seed Pudding with Fresh Berries	Mediterranean Couscous Salad	Grilled Salmon with Mango Salsa, Balsamic Glazed Brussels Sprouts	Dark Chocolate Avocado Mousse
2	Almond Butter Banana Smoothie	Spicy Moroccan Chickpea and Lentil Soup	Spinach and Feta Stuffed Chicken Breast, Roasted Cauliflower with Garlic and Lemon	Baked Apples with Cinnamon and Walnuts
3	Greek Yogurt Parfait with Granola and Berries	Quinoa and Vegetable Stir-Fry	Baked Cod with Garlic and Herb Butter, Sweet Potato and Kale Hash	Fruit Salad with Honey-Lime Dressing
4	Apple Cinnamon Overnight Oats	Roasted Red Pepper and Tomato Soup	Herbed Turkey Meatballs with Zucchini Noodles	Almond Flour Blueberry Muffins
5	Chia Seed Pudding with Fresh Berries	Shrimp and Avocado Salad with Lime Dressing	Chicken and Zucchini Skillet with Garlic and Lemon	Dark Chocolate Avocado Mousse
6	Almond Butter Banana Smoothie	Curried Lentil and Sweet Potato Stew	Mediterranean Tuna Salad	Baked Apples with Cinnamon and Walnuts
7	Greek Yogurt Parfait with Granola and Berries	Mediterranean Couscous Salad	Balsamic Glazed Pork Tenderloin, Eggplant	Chia Seed Pudding with Fresh Berries

			Caponata	
8	Apple Cinnamon Overnight Oats	Spicy Quinoa and Black Bean Stuffed Peppers	Grilled Salmon with Mango Salsa, Balsamic Glazed Brussels Sprouts	Fruit Salad with Honey-Lime Dressing
9	Chia Seed Pudding with Fresh Berries	Creamy Tomato and Basil Soup	Spinach and Feta Stuffed Chicken Breast, Roasted Cauliflower with Garlic and Lemon	Almond Flour Blueberry Muffins
10	Almond Butter Banana Smoothie	Shrimp and Avocado Salad with Lime Dressing	Baked Cod with Garlic and Herb Butter, Sweet Potato and Kale Hash	Dark Chocolate Avocado Mousse
11	Greek Yogurt Parfait with Granola and Berries	Quinoa and Vegetable Stir-Fry	Herbed Turkey Meatballs with Zucchini Noodles	Baked Apples with Cinnamon and Walnuts
12	Apple Cinnamon Overnight Oats	Spicy Moroccan Chickpea and Lentil Soup	Chicken and Zucchini Skillet with Garlic and Lemon	Chia Seed Pudding with Fresh Berries
13	Chia Seed Pudding with Fresh Berries	Mediterranean Couscous Salad	Grilled Salmon with Mango Salsa, Roasted Cauliflower with Garlic and Lemon	Fruit Salad with Honey-Lime Dressing
14	Almond Butter Banana Smoothie	Curried Lentil and Sweet Potato Stew	Balsamic Glazed Pork Tenderloin, Eggplant Caponata	Almond Flour Blueberry Muffins
15	Greek Yogurt Parfait with Granola and Berries	Shrimp and Avocado Salad with Lime Dressing	Spinach and Feta Stuffed Chicken Breast, Sweet Potato and Kale Hash	Dark Chocolate Avocado Mousse

16	Apple Cinnamon Overnight Oats	Spicy Quinoa and Black Bean Stuffed Peppers	Baked Cod with Garlic and Herb Butter, Balsamic Glazed Brussels Sprouts	Baked Apples with Cinnamon and Walnuts
17	Chia Seed Pudding with Fresh Berries	Roasted Red Pepper and Tomato Soup	Mediterranean Tuna Salad	Chia Seed Pudding with Fresh Berries
18	Almond Butter Banana Smoothie	Mediterranean Couscous Salad	Herbed Turkey Meatballs with Zucchini Noodles	Fruit Salad with Honey-Lime Dressing
19	Greek Yogurt Parfait with Granola and Berries	Spicy Moroccan Chickpea and Lentil Soup	Chicken and Zucchini Skillet with Garlic and Lemon	Almond Flour Blueberry Muffins
20	Apple Cinnamon Overnight Oats	Creamy Tomato and Basil Soup	Grilled Salmon with Mango Salsa, Sweet Potato and Kale Hash	Dark Chocolate Avocado Mousse
21	Chia Seed Pudding with Fresh Berries	Shrimp and Avocado Salad with Lime Dressing	Balsamic Glazed Pork Tenderloin, Roasted Cauliflower with Garlic and Lemon	Baked Apples with Cinnamon and Walnuts
22	Almond Butter Banana Smoothie	Quinoa and Vegetable Stir-Fry	Spinach and Feta Stuffed Chicken Breast, Eggplant Caponata	Chia Seed Pudding with Fresh Berries
23	Greek Yogurt Parfait with Granola and Berries	Curried Lentil and Sweet Potato Stew	Baked Cod with Garlic and Herb Butter, Balsamic Glazed Brussels Sprouts	Fruit Salad with Honey-Lime Dressing
24	Apple Cinnamon Overnight Oats	Mediterranean Couscous Salad	Herbed Turkey Meatballs with Zucchini Noodles	Almond Flour Blueberry Muffins

25	Chia Seed Pudding with Fresh Berries	Spicy Quinoa and Black Bean Stuffed Peppers	Chicken and Zucchini Skillet with Garlic and Lemon	Dark Chocolate Avocado Mousse
26	Almond Butter Banana Smoothie	Roasted Red Pepper and Tomato Soup	Grilled Salmon with Mango Salsa, Sweet Potato and Kale Hash	Baked Apples with Cinnamon and Walnuts
27	Greek Yogurt Parfait with Granola and Berries	Spicy Moroccan Chickpea and Lentil Soup	Spinach and Feta Stuffed Chicken Breast, Roasted Cauliflower with Garlic and Lemon	Chia Seed Pudding with Fresh Berries
28	Apple Cinnamon Overnight Oats	Shrimp and Avocado Salad with Lime Dressing	Balsamic Glazed Pork Tenderloin, Eggplant Caponata	Fruit Salad with Honey-Lime Dressing
29	Chia Seed Pudding with Fresh Berries	Creamy Tomato and Basil Soup	Baked Cod with Garlic and Herb Butter, Balsamic Glazed Brussels Sprouts	Almond Flour Blueberry Muffins
30	Almond Butter Banana Smoothie	Mediterranean Couscous Salad	Herbed Turkey Meatballs with Zucchini Noodles	Dark Chocolate Avocado Mousse

CONCLUSION

As we reach the end of this journey through "The Good Energy Cookbook," it's important to reflect on the principles and practices that have guided us toward a healthier, more balanced life. This book has been designed not just as a collection of recipes, but as a comprehensive guide to achieving and maintaining well-being through thoughtful, personalized nutrition and mindful living.

Embracing Holistic Health

We have explored the essentials of an anti-inflammatory and low glycemic diet, delving into how these principles can help reduce chronic inflammation and stabilize blood sugar levels. By focusing on whole, nutrient-dense foods, we've aimed to provide you with recipes that not only nourish your body but also support overall wellness.

Understanding and Using Ingredients Wisely

The chapter on ingredient selection has emphasized the importance of choosing quality, energy-boosting ingredients. Understanding how each ingredient contributes to your health empowers you to make informed choices that align with your personal dietary goals and preferences.

Smart Meal Prep and Planning

Effective meal preparation and planning are key to maintaining a consistent and healthy eating routine. By incorporating the strategies discussed, you can streamline your cooking process, save time, and ensure that you always have nutritious meals ready to support your well-being.

Mindfulness and Eating with Awareness

Mindfulness practices have been highlighted as essential for fostering a deeper connection with your food and yourself. Through mindful eating and stress-reducing techniques, you can enhance your overall health and cultivate a more balanced, fulfilling life.

The Role of Holistic Support

We've examined how a holistic approach to health—encompassing physical, emotional, mental, and spiritual aspects—can create a foundation for lasting well-being. By addressing each of these areas, you can achieve a more integrated and harmonious state of health.

Personalized Nutrition with CGM

Finally, the introduction of Continuous Glucose Monitoring (CGM) has provided a cutting-edge method for personalizing your diet based on real-time glucose data. This technology allows you to tailor your nutritional choices to your unique physiological needs, optimizing your health and well-being in a precise and informed manner.

Moving Forward

As you conclude this book and embark on your journey toward better health, remember that the path to well-being is ongoing and evolving. Use the knowledge and tools provided here to make choices that align with your goals and values. Continue to explore, experiment, and refine your approach to nutrition and self-care.

Remember that achieving and maintaining good health is not about perfection but about making consistent, informed choices that support your overall well-being. Embrace the principles and practices shared in this book, and let them guide you toward a vibrant, energized, and balanced life.

Thank you for joining me on this journey. Here's to your continued health and happiness.

Made in the USA
Las Vegas, NV
15 November 2024

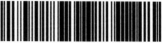

11862509R00077